In Herriot's
SHADOW

Bill Stork, DVM

LITTLE CREEK PRESS®
A DIVISION OF KRISTIN MITCHELL DESIGN, LLC

Mineral Point, Wisconsin USA

Contact Dr. Bill Stork:
Blue Collar Dollar Publishing
author@drbillstork.com
Appearances, online ordering and blog at:
www.drbillstork.com

Library of Congress Control Number: 2014949684

ISBN-10: 0989978443
ISBN-13: 978-0-9899784-4-6

Dedication

Woven throughout this book you will find multiple attempts to erode the concept of the often misguided, "first impression." In doing so you will find your mind liberated to the notion that most people are inherently good. In that respect this book is dedicated to my Mother, Alma Ann Stork.

You will find multiple references to the rewards of productivity, hard work, and respect for the working man. These pages are underpinned by a priority of *family comes first:* an example demonstrated daily and without exception by my dad. Therefore this book is dedicated to my Dad, Bill Stork.

Linda,

thank you so

much.

Peace, Dr. Bill

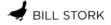 BILL STORK

Table of Contents

BILL STORK

BILL STORK

Family Times

Cat's in the Cradle

"Respect is earned, never given."

"You can work hard enough to overcome what you may lack in intelligence, but you can't be smart enough to overcome being lazy."

I could fill 16 pages of the newspaper with words of wisdom from my dad. I could recite them word for word, punctuation, intonation and pauses, based on the way he inhaled and the context of the situation. Words that elicited an eye roll to a 12-year-old boy have become inarguable, universally applicable truths to a 46-year-old father of two.

As priceless as his words are, it was his actions that are defining. I never had to worry where my dad was. He was either providing for his family or with us.

I recall an evening in the summer of 1978. Mom had prepared the only meal in all my childhood I did not care for — stuffed green peppers. I was still struggling with the first half when the peach-colored, rotary phone on the wall rang. My mom answered, and handed the phone to my dad. In the 5-minute conversation there was mostly listening, a few grunts, three "uh huhs." and it ended with, "I appreciate the offer, but I have a young boy at home."

It took several years to piece things together. It was the Alaskan Pipeline calling. My dad was a heavy equipment operator. Working on the pipeline was like starting as quarterback in the Super Bowl, and could wipe out the family debt in six months.

On Father's Day, there will be cards, hugs, mugs and grilling utensils handed out in appreciation, "for all you do." Somewhere during the course of the day let us all step aside, think hard, and make sure we are being the example of the people we hope our kids will become.

Not to mention, someday, they may have to help change OUR diapers.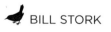

BILL STORK

Q

Tom excused himself to deliver a Natural Light to the gentleman curiously sporting a navy blue blazer and wingtips, playing machines in the corner. Eight notes from an acoustic guitar reverberated through the crowd scattered in small groups around high tops, pool tables, and bar stools in the repurposed pharmacy where I met my cousin for our annual Thanksgiving reconnect.

By the time, "The preacher man says it's the end of time, and the Mississippi River is a goin' dry," every head and shoulders in the Bourbon Barrel rocked, barely perceptibly, on the plodding bass line. Like so many redneck ventriloquists, lips didn't move, but by the time "we say grace, and we say ma'am," the cavernous cinderblock room hummed in the harmony of solidarity.

I sat inexplicably slack-jawed and numb. Careful not to look down, or else explain the tear that rested in my left eyelid.

It was the last act of a day that began wedged between a concrete wall and the prolapsed uterus of a Holstein; 21 hours, 270 miles, a gallon of coffee and two pale ales ago. It was little surprise that at 8:00 a.m. Thanksgiving morning, as I struggled to focus on the Decatur Herald, "they came from the West Virginia coal mines and the Rocky Mountains..." echoed through my head. In short order and a half cup of Folger's from a Lakeview High School mug, Hank Jr. would fade to silent.

As the sun set over the endless horizon of barren Illinois beanfields and wind turbines, Sheila and I headed north. What I could not shake, having nothing to do with turkey and pie, was a distinct sense of missing, and a ten-pound tug at the root of my mesentery. Even the pain of a Packers Thanksgiving Day no-show on national TV should not have tarnished the feel-good of a rare day with our dear family. Sheila settled in for a 200-mile nap, and Remmi and Token sighed. Just past mile marker 65 on I-39N, Hank was back. His bourbon-barrel baritone echoed through a cavernous void in my soul.

"I had a friend from New York City, he never called me by my name, just hillbilly."

With that line, I was back on the shore of Lake Decatur in 1983, six-pound monofilament line on an ultra-light Zebco, with a wad of alfalfa bait wrapped around a treble hook, sitting second stump to the president and founder of the Decatur Carp Club.

Doug Quintenz, "Q." was well over six feet tall, with long blond hair and some variation of a goatee. Trade his work boots for sandals, flannel for a white robe and his Red Man hat for a crown of thorns, and he would be a dead ringer for Jesus Christ himself. That said, in the traditional sense, a saint Doug was not. What I did to bank enough trust with my parents to hang out with Doug, I have not a clue.

Q was the "Master Baiter." to whose skill I aspired when we met at Dave's Tackle Box, on the corner of Nelson Park across from the first Dairy Queen in the world to dump old candy into a cup of ice cream. He was an all-state linebacker at St. Theresa High School — farm boy strong, fearless and fleet of foot. One afternoon a young boy short on allowance money and bluegill decided to help himself to a new rod and reel. To be sporting, Q gave him a head start the width of the parking lot and took a sip of his RC cola, before launching. In minutes, the 6th grader was kicking, crying and apologizing, begging us not to call the cops or tell his mom.

The Decatur Carp Club met regularly on the shores of Lake Decatur and around farm ponds after the Tackle Box closed at 8:00. We had a Mission Statement, firmly enforced, and an elected set of officers. What the meetings of DCC were lacking in Parliamentary Procedure, we more than made up in chewing tobacco and Budweiser.

After graduating from high school in 1981, Doug's foray into higher education was short-lived. Regardless of his ability to crunch running backs and sack quarterbacks, administrators in the eighties had minimal tolerance for student athletes driving their cars through women's dorms. Shortly after the second such incident, he was unceremoniously asked to leave.

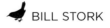 BILL STORK

Back home, his life lacked direction. A brighter man has never been born. Regrettably, common sense doesn't count when an officer is asking you to walk a straight line and touch your nose.

If it is true that "no man stands so tall, as when he stoops to help a child," then Q was 10 foot 2. He had fists that would lay a man stone cold for disrespecting a woman he had never met, and hands that would cradle a baby, kitten or pup. It was of little surprise to those who loved him that a revelation came, the day he learned he was to be a father.

Saturday night bar stools became Sunday morning church pews. He put down the beer cans and picked up hammer, pliers and #16 wire to build a fence for his wife's horse and daughter's pony. Each morning his family joined hands to give thanks for the eggs harvested from the coop out back.

When I last visited, we laughed as he and his son recalled trips to the emergency room. Cuts and bruises were the inevitable consequences of being related to his father. I spoke with his wife as Q read bedtime stories, without mention of the past. As I left, he hugged me, blessed me, and told me that he loved me.

It is with regret that I did not keep contact with Doug. Before his son would graduate high school, his wife would leave him. Too many years of smoking and sedentary living ended his life before he was 50. I will never forget his wisdom, "Willy, everything I own is for sale, just name a price," or "I'm in no shape to start exercising now."

I am obligated to teach my kids to never judge a man with a cigarette on his lips. To live in the hearts of those we leave behind, is not to die. I knew "Q." and a country boy can survive. ❧

A Tail of Destruction

Margie was 23 pounds of tongue, tail and adorable. She had been with her family for two weeks, had not had an accident in six days, was comfortable in the crate and slept through the night without making a sound. She was charming beyond words, at ease with a crowd and easily self-entertained. Whether meeting a German Shepherd or Jack Russell Terrier, she approached with a play bow and a precocious sideways "woof?"

As we made conversation, I carefully checked for bite abnormalities, heart murmurs, hernias and conformation. The 12x12 exam room could barely contain the feel-good as Margie politely sat for treats, took them gently, then extended her paw to ask for another. Megan, our technician, confirmed her birthday as August 15. As we speculated on her breeding, I watched her 12-inch tail wag the entire Margie, from her ears south. At only 90 days of age, her hinder stood close to 10 inches off the ground. The engaging personality, the soft, wiry coat, long snout and friendly tongue, and The Tail...

The warm fuzzies were sucked under the door as déjà vu flooded the tiny space. My fading Texas tan turned to ashen. As Megan deftly knelt to collect a kiss and deliver a belly rub, I foresaw that the years to follow were sure to be filled with love and laughter. Equally certain, there would be damage deposits, destruction and pain.

My veterinary career began at age 14, working for Dr. Bill Van Alstine at the Brush College Animal Hospital. Doc V was known for his heart, handshake and mustache. It was equally true that he was not of the nature to turn his back on a dollar. Being the youngest, least qualified and the last hired, I was in charge of cleaning up after and walking the dogs and cats he boarded on weekends and holidays.

BCAH had 6 runs, 18 cages, three bathrooms, an office, two exam rooms, a surgery and two hallways. On many a Christmas Eve, Thanksgiving and Independence Day, the future Dr. Stork was cleaning up after thirty animals, morning, noon and night. By my 30th anniversary of practicing, I hope to have cleaned more anal glands than kennels.

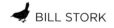 BILL STORK

After three and a half decades, I remember a couple breeds and pooping patterns. One, however, I will never forget. Her name was Bittsy.

Bittsy belonged to our closest family friends, Wayne and Shirley Cox. She was as friendly as a Disney tour guide, with a wiry coat and a long rounded snout. She was 20 inches at the hip, with a tail that could be registered as a lethal weapon. You may soon begin to feel my fear.

(At this point, a pause. Recall Dr. Stork's "rough math" when telling stories: numbers are generally rounded to the nearest "5" or "10." for the sake of easier figuring. Mostly, they are rounded down, in the event they should be challenged. Occasionally they are rounded up, if they do not seem sufficiently dramatic to carry a story. Construction-based stories are reported in English measurements. Science and medical stories are based in metric.)

Bittsy's tail measured 26 inches long (the metric system hadn't made it to the States yet). Using water displacement and tissue density data, we concluded it must weigh about 3.5 lbs. While wagging at a constant rate of 30 rpm, with surges up to 60, the velocity of her tail tip could top out at 55mph, and was capable of delivering a blow roughly equivalent to that of the burly kid who always hit the homerun in 7th grade whiffle ball.

This was an absolutely life-altering realization for the Cox family.

They would learn to adapt. Like the "Screamin' Eagle" at Six Flags, there was a taped line on the frame of the door. No children below this line were to be left unattended, as the risk of concussion was equal to that of tackle football or Bantam level youth hockey. Nothing of value, liquids or food capable of staining was to ever be placed on a coffee table. As adorable as she was, her name was never to be called unless she was outdoors.

The Cox family took a California vacation, leaving Bittsy at BCAH for the 10 days they were gone.

Checkbook open, pen in hand, Shirley arrived to pick up Bittsy.

The consummately professional receptionist, Adele, slid the neatly typed invoice across the counter. Shirley's eyes drifted straight to the bottom line: $3,500.25.

"SAY WHAT?!"

Boarding, bedding, food and bath were the standard $55.00.

The balance included drywall patches, trim boards dislodged from door frames, broken panes of glass, and hockey goalie shin pads. Also itemized were radiograph and replacement of dislocated knee-cap prior to hockey pads, as well as ice packs and aspirin for Dr. Van Alstine, whose waist was but a few inches above the tip of Bittsy's tail.

The future of health care is anyone's guess, but some things are a dead lock cinch. For Margie's family, the future is full of licks, laughs and love. There will also be plenty of broken glass and spilled milk. ❧

 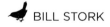

Git-R-Done

As we approach Labor Day, the weeks become a tribute to the working men and women of our country.

I have no problem with Larry the Cable Guy making millions off the blue collar battle cry, Git-R-Done. What's regrettable is that we've managed to stray far from the mentality that gave birth to his little tag line.

Where I come from, Git 'er Done applies to a job, in a place and time. It is assumed more often than spoken. When it is spoken, it comes from the back of the throat, through clenched teeth and finishes with a slight tick of the head. It starts the motion toward a job you may have done a hundred times, or never at all. It also starts with an assumption: whatever "it" is, it will get done.

It will get done with whatever you have, whomever you have to help, and regardless of snow, wind or rain.

Git 'er Done is growled by men and women who build stuff, fix stuff and grow stuff. When they are done they don't fist bump and high-five. They pack up, go home and do it again the next day.

These are the folks for whom Labor Day was begun, and we thank you. ❧

Little Red Iron Horse

The year was 1977.

It was the best of times: Saturday Night Fever, Barry Manilow, Jimmy Carter, the first female Episcopalian minister.

It was the worst of times: we lost Groucho Marx, Steve Bilko and Elvis Presley.

At least as momentous was mechanization of the first business I would be involved in. I had been mowing five lawns and shoveling snow for a few years. Market research suggested there were opportunities for expansion. So a meeting was called among the rank and file, accounting, and mechanical shop (meaning, Mom and Dad and I talked about it at supper one night). We would expand our fleet from a self-propelled Toro and two snow shovels to include a riding lawn tractor.

It has been said, with accuracy, that a Stork and his dollar do not easily part. Though everything at 1195 Nickey Avenue performed its function and worked when you needed it, we were never the first owner. So it would have been totally out of character and over budget to march in to the local John Deere store and arrange a payment plan for a brand-new green machine.

Dad always traded trucks and cars on the coldest day of the year, and negotiated in the parking lot. So, in character and out of season we scoured classified ads and auctions, and bought two tractors. The first was a 1965 Wheel Horse, with a blown motor, but a brand-new hydrostatic transmission. The other wasn't nearly as new, but had a rebuilt 12hp Kohler. So, over several nights in the early winter 1977, Mom was thanked for dinner, dishes were cleared, and Dad and I headed to the garage.

That garage was a 20x28, tongue-and-groove temple to Midwestern work ethic and family values, and was roofed in one day. My dad, our cousin and I were stripping and shingling when Carl Eads, the union steward from the Clinton Nuclear Power Plant called. A man hadn't shown, and a machine sat idle. Cousin Jim thought that would be a good time for a glass of iced tea and a break; I

 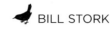 BILL STORK

thought that if Dad was going to work and provide for his family, he wasn't going to have to come home and put a roof on the garage as well. So we put the hammer (and the chalk line) down. When Dad came home, we were putting the ladders away.

The garage had no name like "The Hub" or "Man Cave," no beer fridge, and no TV.

Location and orientation to the house was crucial for maximum production. Initially, Dad espoused the value of a detached garage: "An attached garage is so warm, it'll rust your car out." Later (out of Mom's earshot), he added that the 50 feet between the back door and the garage was just enough of an impediment to reduce interruptions. It was wired with three-phase to run the welder and a propane tank to run the bullet heater. A telephone, on the other hand, was conspicuously absent. Same notion.

Long before Jiffy Lube and spreadsheets, the maintenance record of every car, lawn mower and truck was logged in magic marker between the studs, "77 Merc, OLF, 81,500 miles, 1-5-81." This was no ten-minute oil change: every grease zerk would be over full, every bearing and linkage inspected, and the next entry would be well before 83,000 miles.

Never mind the manufacturer's recommendation. The cars in this garage were paid for up front with blue collar dollars and they transported his family.

The only new things in the garage were Father's Day and Christmas presents.

Along with Charlie Rich, Glenn Campbell and Kenny Rogers, the shop radio — frozen by decades of dust on WSOY AM — played "One Piece at a Time."

Not dissimilar to Johnny's Cadillac, we put together the functional parts of the two ten-year-old mini-tractors, and in no time, she was running. If Johnny's Caddy ran like a song, this was more like a blues tune. With a three-foot snowplow, a hunk of #9 wire, some strap steel and the welder from my uncle's farm, we had a fully articulating, three-angle blade; though we did have to cut a half moon out of the lever to accommodate the fly wheel when we angled the snow on Mrs. Hayne's driveway.

Long before front wheel assist, Dad welded two drive gears from a Caterpillar Tournapull to a steel plate to make wheel weights. That, along with tire chains, assured we had all 10.5 horses on the ground. She worked like a dream during the first big snowstorm, but I found myself inhaling exhaust. Dad got to work: a foot of 6-inch steel pipe and a homemade baffle made sure the whole neighborhood knew it was us coming, and put both the exhaust and a plume of blue flame well above my head when I got after the big drifts.

Dad worked construction. He could drown out the Civil War with his snoring, but when the first snowflake fluttered onto one of the 21 white pines outside his window, he was up and at 'em. While his truck warmed and coffee brewed, he would train a 250-watt flood lamp on the oil pan of my little tractor. She could push a mountain of snow, but the cold-blooded little cast iron Kohler was not about to turn over when it was below 15F.

By the time he got to work, there would be a couple of inches on the ground. Like a blue collar ballet, Dad ran a 30-year-old Caterpillar road grader and his buddy, Gene Prasun*, ran a Bobcat Skid loader. They would clear the parking lots of grocery stores, churches and hospitals, while I headed out on my 12-horse lawn tractor to clear the neighbors' driveways.

*During a historic blizzard in 1978 that dumped 21 inches of snow, Dad and Gene had been plowing for nearly 30 straight hours. Dad was pulling a healthy drift away from the curb at the Piggly Wiggly, when a Crown Victoria slipped around his road grader and parked right in front of the machine. The driver leapt out, removed his glove and gestured to Dad in a fashion that was less than appreciative, and went inside.

Rather than fuss, and without so much as eye contact, Gene slipped the bucket of his Bobcat under the bumper of the Ford Sedan and lifted it off the ground. Dad

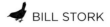 BILL STORK

passed with the grader and meticulously deposited several tons of slush and snow neatly under the car from stern to bow.

Gene gently let the front end down and circled to the back. By the time the driver had returned with his emergency 2:00 a.m. carton of Camels, Gene had surgically removed the excess snow from the doors. The driver would hop in and put it in drive, but the car would go nowhere for several days, as the wheels were 4 inches off the ground.

I once saw a sign at Denver International Airport: "The top 10 professions of 2025 don't exist yet."

As the father of a 10- and 12-year-old, I would have been stopped dead in my tracks, but I was on a moving walkway. For two years I have contemplated how to help my kids prepare. In the meantime, what I have come to realize is that I don't remember how much money I made plowing snow when I was a kid.

What I do remember is that I did it with a machine built from scrap iron and spare parts, in the garage, with my dad. I would like to tell you that it never broke down, but when it did I was obsessed with cobbling it back together, so that when dad came home from plowing his parking lots, my driveways were clean. Mr. Carter was the fire chief. Mr. Shemanski had a heart attack; Mr. Funk a stroke. They were doing well, but, just in case, an ambulance had to get in.

I vividly recall plowing from home to the farthest customer. There is no forgetting the feeling of driving past 17 driveways void of a single snowflake, winged wide for easy entrance and exit, and sidewalks shoveled for safety.

We are marching deeper into the age of technology and further from the age of production. In 2012, a mere 1% of our population claimed agriculture as their main source of income. Inevitable as it may be, I'm not in the least bit comfortable.

Including me, let us not deprive our children and ourselves the opportunity of physical accomplishment; to know the visceral satisfaction of having built something, fixed something, moved something, or grown something. And, if all goes well, we might give our children an opportunity to help a neighbor and a gain a healthy measure of respect for people who do it daily. ❧

BILL STORK

The Garage

Dad claimed no expertise as a carpenter. For that matter, even though his body of work ranged from nuclear power plants to overpasses, and he fixed anything from Caterpillar D8 bulldozers to leaky faucets, Dad claimed expertise of no kind.

"Just shut your mouth and do your work. If you're worth a (vernacular), folks will know it."

What can be said is everything he ever built is still standing, aesthetics notwithstanding. The extra eight feet in the garage would make room for the workbench, welding and fabrication shop, parts, and hardware. The bench was behind where we parked the truck. Long before ergonomics, it was just above waist high, secured to the wall and the foundation, and he probably sent an anchor down to bedrock. Just so if you had to break loose a rusty bolt with a "cheater" clamped in the vise that had once stood in his uncle's machine shop, you knew it wouldn't go anywhere.

On the back wall of the garage were 64 bins full of every size nut, bolt, screw and pin that had ever been thrown away or salvaged. In their first life, they were scoops from a grain elevator at Archer Daniels Midland. You learned in a hurry to check the bolt bin first, then drill your hole.

Cordless hand tools were two decades in the future. By my recollection, every drill and grinder cord in the shop had been spliced and soldered back together, including the Black and Decker 1/4 inch utility drill, made in Towson, MO, USA. You could work in the dark if you needed to because it shot sparks six inches out of the housing, but you never had to look for the chuck. It was circumferentially secured with black electrical tape, halfway up the cord.

A big hand-held grinder that would eat your lunch (and your favorite Decatur Carp Club T-shirt) if you didn't hold on tightly had been rescued from a dumpster at the Clinton Nuclear Power Plant. If the power ever went out, we could run a spliced, salvaged extension cord to the neighbors. If you needed a grinder and a drill on the same job, you could plug them into the same cord — Dad had spliced two female ends on a couple of the cords.

On the north was an open-sided extension we called the lean-to. When I got my driver's license, it would protect my 1974 Plymouth Valiant. Slant 6, 4-door, vinyl seats and AM radio: look out girls, here I come.

Before that, it protected our 14-foot Feathercraft fishing boat, and the tractor fit nicely behind. My dad, grandpa and I caught a lot of fish out of that boat. You just couldn't be in a hurry or afraid to get your feet wet. Grandpa had encountered a rock in Rice Lake, Wisconsin, and punched a pretty good hole in the bottom. Dad pounded that out with a rubber mallet, cut a piece of scrap aluminum to cover the hole, riveted and sealed it down.

The boat was pushed around by a 9-1/2 Horse Johnson that always started on the third pull; never the first or second. This, despite the fact we bought it for cheap. It had been given up for dead, having spent a few days on the bottom of Lake Sarah.

On the back corner was the storage shed. Nearly half the space was taken up by racks full of scrap lumber and steel. The rest held our push mower, rakes and hand tools.

Just inside the door was a five gallon bucket full of used motor oil. That's where the shovels and hoes were kept. Dirt was scraped off after every use, and the cuttin' edge touched up on the grinder. If I had whiskers, I could have shaved with the spade.

Underground parking at a condominium will keep the rain and snow off your windshield and prevent the sun from fading the paint of your Porsche. In a garage, a young boy comes to understand, firsthand, the difference between "wants" and "needs." He learns to make do with what he has, and take care of it. ❧

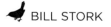 BILL STORK

Fishin' Magician

Many things have been said of my dad. Among the truest was summed up by his childhood friend and fellow Seabee, Leroy the one-eyed mechanic, "Stork, I could give you a brand new Rolls Royce and in three days you'd have something homemade hangin' off the dashboard."

For the sake of clarity and in defense of the old man, there are some things you need to know about his inventions. They are without fail highly functional and ruggedly constructed, if not indestructible. His designs were ergonomic long before Detroit, though aesthetics have been variable at best.

Research, design, and engineering take place with a pencil, sharpened with a pocket knife, on the back of whatever happens to be lying on the work bench. Raw materials often include scraps of PVC, angle iron, battery straps and hose. Wood is a last option. Though creative, Dad is not a finish carpenter, and you can't weld plywood. To start with new parts would be to spend money. Unless it involves helping his son through college or taking his wife on vacation, that's just not likely.

It has been said that many great inventions are the product of necessity. That would certainly hold true when Dad's best fishing buddy and cousin suffered a massive heart attack a few years, and several fish frys ago. Forty-five minutes after receiving the call, Dad was at Springfield Memorial Hospital with a Stanley thermos and paperback Louis L'Amour. Over the next three days our family cycled through the waiting room, but Dad stood vigil.

Cousin Harry had suffered a massive heart attack and survival was anything but certain. Clots had lodged in several of the great coronary arteries, his arm and his brain. He awoke from the coma 72 hours later, minus his right arm and short term memory; sense of humor intact.

Noting the empty sleeve of his hospital gown, Harry's first words were "Darn, now I'm gonna have to figure out how to pee with my left hand."

Without a word (or a nap), Dad left Harry to work on that, and beat a path back to his garage. A man who'd just lost his arm, and nearly his life, needed a light at the end of the tunnel.

Three days in a hospital waiting room gives a retired construction worker a lot of time to design innovative fishing gear. Dad liberated two straps from an old ski vest, cut a piece of scrap PVC in a 1/3 circle, and padded the underside with shelving rubber.

A modified Berkley fishing rod holder and an alligator clamp would render a one-handed crappie fisherman fully functional: perfectly capable of tying hooks, casting, reeling and landing anything that bit.

Once able to secure the device to his own leg with one hand, Dad headed back to Springfield Memorial Hospital, cardiac ICU.

For those in search of tangible evidence of a superior being, I present Exhibit A: If Harry'd had a different cousin and fishin' buddy, he'd be on dry land, eating Mrs. Paul's Frozen Fish Parts.

If Dad had a different fishing partner, he may be on the bottom of the lake.

Ironic as it may seem, for a man whose first love after family is fishing, Dad swims like the cast-iron flywheel off a John Deere. He also enjoys telling a good story. To the point that, on the 4th or 5th re-telling, fishing buddies not named Harry Nichols have threatened to throw him overboard.

Having a one-armed fishing partner with short-term memory loss makes for a perfect day on the lake. ◈

 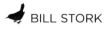 BILL STORK

Up Nort'

After nearly 20 years in this great state, I've finally figured it out. As I sip a Rocky's Revenge, on the shore of a lake I don't even know the name of, the sun sets over a two-log fire. Calvin casts and his bobber settles into the ripple. Paige, cross-legged in a wooden Adirondack, intently absorbs the next page of "The Kite Runner." Sheila, a spittin' image, silently reflects on 37 years with her 96-year-old grandma. A smile creases her temple as Remmi and Token dock dive and race for a smooth piece of driftwood.

This is "Up North."

Not because ice out was only six weeks ago and I could hear a bear fart in the UP from where I sit, but because the cellphone is in the cabin and my concerns south of Portage.

Next week, our lives will be dictated by soccer coaches, limping Labradors, and accounts receivable. Times like these will happen only when we recognize their necessity and make them. When they do, let's exorcise extemporaneous thoughts and internalize every beauty the moments have to offer.

Realizing it's more about who you are with than where you are, I can think of nowhere else I'd rather be than right here in Wisconsin. After all, for folks from the Flatland, we live Up North. ❧

Up Nort', the Sequel

Revelations from the river side... Everybody has limitations — whether it be lack of intelligence, or having only one hand. As for those who think they're perfect, they have the greatest disability of all.

In a recent *Non Sequitur,* Danae and her talking Pygmy Clydesdale, Lucy, were on an adventure. It was the first day of summer vacation and Lucy led the way. "Where are we going?" Danae asked, head buried in her phone, checking her Facebook newsfeed. "We'll know when we get there," Lucy trudged on. In the next panel, Danae stopped cold. "Hey, I lost reception!" "We're here," declared Lucy.

Let the record show that most, if not all, things are relative, not the least of which is the mystical location, "Up North." I have friends from Rockford who treasure their time on Rock Lake, and family who farm near Fort, and escape to a trailer and campfire on the Wisconsin River, near Portage. Most recently for me it was an hour and a half north of the world's greatest pie, just off state highway 27.

Regardless of coordinates on the Gazetteer, "Up North" is where your biggest concern becomes spinners or surface bait, and whether to pack rain gear, sunscreen, or both. Packing industrial strength 95% DEET is simply survival (although do not spray it on the paint on your car, or on yourself if you are pregnant, immune-compromised or elderly).

On rare occasions, the "sometime you oughta, you're more than welcome, well I'm gonna do that" conversations over a picnic table at a family gathering come to fruition. On this occasion, my functional brother-in-law invited us to join a 20-year tradition of fishing on the Flambeau Flowage.

My dad has fished for 65 years, in seven states, on ten different lakes. Always for crappie, from the security of his 16-foot floating museum of mechanic's aftermarket modifications. On the stand next to his throne, the articles in Outdoor Life about smallmouth

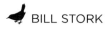 BILL STORK

bass fishing are dog-eared and worn thin. Though Dad has spent the bulk of his retirement on the water, and four years in the United States Navy, he swims like a cinder block.

On the Flambeau Flowage, the river flows fast at times, and they fish from canoes. Days shy of Dad's birthday number 79, I figured I might try and take a few days off. When my 15-year-old son said sure, he'd like to come as well, the decision was made.

Much is made of the romance of fishing, and for good reason. You are never so aware of your place in life until the next generation is in the bow of your canoe, and the previous generation upstream 25 yards.

You could hear Dad's war whoops from Cadott to Hayward as his rod tip tickled his knuckles and he reeled furiously. "Hey, Calvin!" he bellowed, as he held a 4 lb "smallie" for us to see.

Meanwhile, I asked Calvin to put down his pole and pick up a paddle. We rowed furiously cross-current and downwind to nose into a shallow, grassy pool on the downstream side of an island where there should be fish. I dropped anchor, planted my paddle and locked my jaw, fighting to keep the boat in perfect position. Calvin tossed his homemade popper deep in an eddy pool.

As the rings spread, I found myself trembling. Time on Earth is finite, and ten minutes previous my heart had soared as Dad checked one off the proverbial bucket list. Right then and there, I found myself summoning every source of strength and fortune, focused and hoping with all I had that the water would boil, the bait would disappear, and my boy — three years from college and rapidly becoming a man — would catch a fish.

Praying hard to share the experience, at that moment, more than I ever had, I understood the length, depth and breadth of a father's love for his child. ◆

Give It All You Got

I feel sorry for my son, trapped in a car with a contemplative father. We've just returned from scenic Rice Lake, Wisconsin, home of the 2012 Bantam 2A State Boys Hockey Tournament.

Calvin is a smart, strong and skilled hockey player. Regrettably, this weekend three other teams were eight goals smarter, stronger and faster. The NCAA mantra, "99% of student athletes will go professional, in something else," comes to mind.

Strong on his skates and a stout defender, for five periods if you wanted to get a puck past #93, you had to buy it. Then came a 15-minute power failure. Dad can barely stand up on skates, and will never criticize a hockey mistake. What I have no tolerance for is lack of effort.

As Calvin watched two Wausau Warjacks fly past, he stood flat-footed as a puck — like a softball in a Wednesday night beer league — dribbled past. The goalie he's charged to protect crouched and spread. In two uncontested passes, the puck slammed past the goalie's right ear, top shelf.

We are obligated, as Teddy Roosevelt (approximately) said, to do the best we can, with what we've got, where we are, when we're there. Dr. Stork would follow that we must prepare our bodies and minds as best we can. Whether racing your bike in Badger State Games, or extracting a deformed calf, when you find yourself maxed out: embrace it. Then, go beyond.

When family, teammates or animals put faith in us, IF we do as above, we can never truly lose. We can accept the outcome, learn from it, and get better.

Having been a kid once, I can only imagine being captive in a Chevy Trailblazer for 237 miles. Looking to contain the lecture, I said my piece, and bought Shamrock shakes. At mile 164, we passed a yellow VW bug, he double-punched me in the right arm, and we got back to normal. ❖

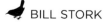 BILL STORK

Blue Moon of Kentucky

I stepped outside to experience 80 degrees and green grass in March. I returned minutes later with that, and so much more.

Two of our favorite people, Don and Mary Grant, were doing the same. We exchanged the obvious weather comments, then Don pulled me aside.

"You know, Doc, I really enjoy your articles, but especially the humanity they often display."

While we appreciate and are motivated by every compliment, this one set off a series of thoughts. In the 20 feet from the blacktop to the front door I had a first time realization, a hearty appreciation, and a mission.

I realized it is the humanity that I appreciated in *The Waltons*. Every Thursday night our family would share a bowl of popcorn. After Maw and Paw said their goodnights, John Boy would reflect on people and events that moved him. It is the beauty of the folks in Northern Wisconsin that Mike Perry captures brilliantly in *Population 485**. It is the way I see the world, and what motivated me to become a veterinarian and eventually put pen to paper. It has been nurtured by people like The Amazing Dick Bass and Kishan Khemani.

However, the notion that all people are inherently good was first demonstrated to me by Alma Ann Beasley.

Through Alma Ann Beasley's big brown eyes and bifocals, there were only good people. She did not see people as dressed in the finest apparel or a 30-year-old flannel. She didn't know black, white, straight or gay. She didn't acknowledge whether people were decorated by degrees, or by calluses, grease and scars.

Ann was incapable of putting herself first. It was once said, with little exaggeration, that if a neighbor fell ill the paramedics would have to politely ask her to step aside. She would be there — with a hot casserole, a bouquet of flowers and a pitcher of iced tea.

A friend in need was a failure of sorts. For someone to ask for help would be to risk spending an ounce of pride or dignity — she was there first. Though she may have tipped the scale at 120 lbs, at least half must have been heart. If she had the strength in her body to help, she would. If she didn't, she would recruit.

Ann would be the first to tell you there is no shortage of good people in this world. What made her special was that the list of those she cared about was in no way limited to those who were kind by nature.

Twelve grit surly and downright disagreeable were no deterrent to Ann. Anger and outward hostility were red flags and flashing lights; a sure sign of soul who needed to be heard, understood and embraced. While it is certain she would never harbor a negative thought or utter an ill word about another human being, it was not good enough. She was first to help, so that no one else would think or speak badly of the person.

So Don, I thank you. I can imagine no greater gift than the recognition of humanity. To fully understand that we can all grow from, and give back to every human interaction is to find yourself always surrounded by great people, whether that be with those with whom we are in lock-step, or those we oppose.

For that I can take no credit and give all thanks to Alma Ann Beasley, my mom. Though dementia slowly took her mind, it could not touch her spirit. Her toe never failed to tap at the sound of Bill Monroe, and the last words she spoke, were Thank You.

As a mother's day gift, I offer these words. In doing so, I obligate myself to do unto others as she did, and so her grandchildren may know her better. If another parent should read these words and be moved to recall the examples set by those they admire, all the better.

Happy Mother's Day. I Love You, I miss you, I'm trying.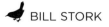

In the Name of the Father

On May 16, 2020, there will be a party. I'm not in the least bit concerned what day of the week it may fall on, but on that day I will declare myself a Cheesehead and a card-carrying Packers fan. Then I will have spent more than half my life in the great state of Wisconsin, among some of the finest people on Earth.

That said, I make no attempt to diminish my country of origin: Decatur, Illinois. We are referred to in terms both endearing, and not so. The one more neutral, and inarguable by virtue of its accuracy, is "Flatlander."

I will offer that, while not striking topographically, those flat lands are the most productive in the world. While traveling south on I-39, imagine that occasionally the rain must fall. When it does, water the corn can't absorb makes its way through field tiles, drainage ditches and eventually creeks (we say cricks). When hundreds of those cricks flow to the center of Moultrie County, they become the Kaskaskia River.

As I climb out of the Kishwaukee River Valley, the skies open. Breaths come more easily and I lose all sense of encumbrance. It could be that I am an hour closer to my family, or what this land means to me. What the flatlands may lack in topography, we more than compensate for in horizon.

Sunrises and sunsets are a commodity in Illinois. During my adult years in the flatlands I missed few of either, as that would be to live less than the day had to offer. Unobstructed, you can see for two counties in any given direction. As the sun rises, if there are 10 particles of ragweed, dust, fog or frost in the air the light is diffracted into more colors than you will ever find on any flat screen TV.

You will never feel smaller than to watch an approaching thunderstorm devour a clear blue sky. If you are ever fortunate enough to find yourself passing through Macon County, Illinois, at sunset in October, I beg you to pull to the side of the road. If you are to pass a field during soybean harvest at sunset, you will find yourself no less impaired than if you had been drinking fine red wine and texting at the same time.

While Wisconsin is now and will always be the Dairy State, Illinois is made more beautiful by its own productivity. We and our buddies to the left and the right are the breadbasket. If a bushel of corn can feed 50 people for a day, then between every pair of mile markers is enough corn to feed over six million people for a day. From Rockford, Illinois, to Paducah, Kentucky, you will pass 400 such mile markers, and the scene is repeated for the width of Iowa, Illinois, Indiana and Ohio.

Each cluster of grain bins in the distance is a tiny town with a railroad running through. At harvest time, millions of bushels of grain make their way from field to rail cars, to barges on the Mississippi River, downstream to the Gulf of Mexico. As you fly through on cruise control to St. Louis, the endless fields of green outside your air conditioning are feeding the world.

It is around the Kaskaskia that Dad would hold me on his lap while riding motorcycles through the river bottoms and ravines. That is, until September 1970. In order to control flooding of valuable farm land downstream, the U.S. Army Corps of Engineers built a dam, and the Kaskaskia River became Lake Shelbyville.

Dad and I mostly preferred to build things, fix things, and cut firewood. But presented with a lake, there is but one thing to do — fish in it. Lake Shelbyville is a gem: 26 miles long and 11,000 acres with endless coves and tributaries. Towering over the terminus like a beacon is Our Lady of the Immaculate Conception Catholic Church. This was, for the most part, perfect.

By my way of thinking, every day on the lake is great. They can be further subdivided into days when you need to be giving thanks, and days when you could use a little divine intervention in order to fill the fryer. Father's Day 1979 was one of the more fortunate days. By 8:00 Mass our basket was already half full. We anchored our 14-foot Feather Craft with the 9.5 horse Johnson just off shore, and meticulously scrubbed our hands and forearms in the lake, wiping them on the pale red shop towel. Our Levi's would absorb

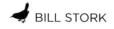 BILL STORK

the excess as we sprinted up the hill and through the door, just in time for opening prayers and welcome.

We had never figured Catholicism as a shirt and tie religion. So long as you were respectful, carrying a bit of guilt and a fiver for the collection, you could pretty much come as you are. As history will show, on this day we pushed a bit.

Attending "Our Lady" was not just about location. The flock was tended by a priest who was as inspirational in his messages as he was physically intimidating. I still recall parts of his sermons to this day. Like Bill Walton in robes, when he spread his arms, he stretched from one altar boy to the other.

The first sign of trouble should have been that we had an entire pew to ourselves. Oblivious, Dad and I were there to give thanks and absorb some inspiration. The gravity of the situation didn't really set in until collection. When we turned to pass the basket, there were two empty rows behind us.

When it was time to offer a handshake, a shoulder clasp and a sign of peace, we must have been surrounded by every hippie in southern Illinois. From a distance, they offered instead peace signs, and a polite, if not sideways nod.

The Catholic service is all about preparing to receive the body and blood of Christ. As we proceeded to the altar for communion, the hippies maintained their buffer zone. I thought it was a perfect day for a "dine and dash" — we could easily have been over the hill and out of sight by the time the congregation got the green light. Instead, head down and hands folded, Dad and I returned to the solitude of our pew.

When Mass was ended, Father Walton didn't have to tell us twice to "go in peace to love and serve the Lord." That is exactly what we attempted to do.

Looking at the floor and hugging the bulletin board, we were nearly past when Father Walton's massive hand wrapped my spindly bicep. There was little room for more fear as he bent down and asked, "Where are they biting?"

Mom had always speculated that Dad's hearing loss was more selective than medical. She may have a case. Two steps ahead, he spun on a dime. Switching from defense to offense faster than a cornerback making an interception, he replied, as I exhaled.

"You have got to be kidding. With or without divine intervention, with feet that size you can walk on water, part the seas, and feed the masses with a loaf of bread and a couple of fish." Surely he took a breath but it didn't seem so.

"Here an old construction worker and his kid catch a few fish, and we've got to tell you where."

Were it not for the upturned corner of his eyes and grin, he may still be saying Our Fathers and Hail Marys.

Father Walton never missed a beat. "Mr. Stork, there is nothing that feels better than to share."

He must have been wearing a flannel shirt under his robes, and had a boat in the water. Twenty minutes later Father Walton, Dad and I were dipping minnows and jigs around the same tree in the mouth of the cove in Sand Creek.

 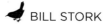

Man vs. Beast

"With beauty that's beyond compare, with flaming locks of auburn hair, with ivory skin and eyes of emerald green," Dolly Parton painted the image of her nemesis.

"Your smile is like a breath of spring, your voice is like a soft summer rain," she begged Jolene not to take her man.

To that description add family values, accountability and the "on-court awareness" of an NBA point guard. Only then do you have an image of a woman whom I respectfully admired, for the better part of 15 years. Proximity and another half-decade have only served to enhance and amplify what I had suspected from afar.

To the women in the audience, I offer the above as a rationalization. To the men, an explanation as to how I came to co-parent a 44 lb cattle dog.

Sheila is the Chief Operating Officer of Wisconsin Equine Clinic and Hospital in Oconomowoc. She is charged with the responsibility of middle-managing a staff of 30 highly skilled, pathologically compassionate horse nuts. Her responsibilities range from payroll to physical plant, and it's not unusual to find her on the business end of a bedding fork stripping stalls at 8 o'clock on a Sunday night.

Evening conversations are motivational, and often filled with superlatives describing the synchrony that pervades her staff. It seems unthinkable that so much as a sliver of compassion fatigue, burn out, or pissed-off should ever creep in. In order to ensure that is the case for years to come, on the insistence of her superiors she will make a semi-annual sojourn to Southwest Wyoming.

On a 12"x12" map, the Woody Bartlett Ranch is about a quarter-inch square. In a 3/4 ton diesel pickup truck pulling a 6-slot horse trailer, it's a three-hour ride on a gravel road and a sore ass. Dr. Bartlett is an 80-year-old, semi-retired veterinarian with three ranches, two airplanes, a girlfriend half his age, and no social filters.

The ranch is run by a crew of cowboys headed up by an Idaho Mormon transplant named Jed Hirschi, and his now-wife Rachel Rose Miller.

Jed is a lariat and spurs cowboy who doesn't own a John Deere Gator, Jeep or ATV. He rides a horse 365 days a year. Jed also reads the Wall Street Journal from cover to cover and treats every foal and calf on the 80,000 acre ranch like it was his first puppy. It is said that behind every good cowboy is a wife that works in town; I beg to differ. There isn't a town to work in, and the Bartlett Ranch would come to a screeching halt without her.

Every spring, 25 to 30 cowboys looking for square meals, a paycheck and couple notches in their belt find their way to the ranch. Two-year-old geldings are rounded from the range and corralled. Seven straight sunrises will find cowboys and horses locked in negotiation. In the name of survival, the scale of mutual respect is tilted — as cowboy looks to earn it from the horse. All in a day's work, 75 horses will be saddled, ridden, groomed and fed.

Shortly after sunset there's chuck-wagon, guitar around the campfire, and shut-eye. Colt Clinic at the Bartlett Ranch is all about saddle-breakin' horses that will make their way to rodeos, barrel-races and fairs from Oregon to Georgia in two weeks' time. Whiskey-drinkin', women, and trucks with big tires is the fictional fodder for so many bubblegum country artists in baseball caps and football stadiums. Occasionally a colt will rear and tear off a cowboy's ear, buying him a ride to Cheyenne and costing a half-day's work. So far nary a broken bone.

I can't begin to imagine the carnage if it weren't for one Rachel. At birth she meets every foal before it hits the ground. First she ensures that he nurses. Then he is haltered, rubbed, injected, conditioned and imprinted on the people he will only see from a distance for the next two years.

To my knowledge she doesn't write songs or sing, but Rachel Rose Miller bears a striking resemblance to Dolly Parton, with no less swagger and class. Whether she's walking down Bowie Avenue in Chugwater, Wyoming or Michigan Avenue in Chicago, she will be noticed.

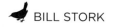 BILL STORK

On October 15, 2009, Sheila had been on the ranch for six days of a three week sabbatical. She lulled me with questions of concern about work, and how were the horses. Proving that is love deaf as well as blind, I did not hear the honey-sweet tone that suggested what was to come.

She had two weeks, and she played me like a fish on a line.

First, she described the litter of puppies who had been born three weeks before she arrived. Like Ray Charles at a demolition derby I asked, "Oh, that sounds cute, how many and what breed are they?"

Deliberately vague, she fed me details, as absence grew the heart fonder. In time we would learn there were nine: mom was an Australian Shepherd and dad was a Blue Heeler, both of whom had been led away by a pack of wolves (true story).

"Beauty that's beyond compare, with flaming locks of auburn hair," Dolly's epic words echoed through my mind.

Love, though deaf and blind, is not completely dumb. Her soft-sell gave me days to think. She could just as easily have asked, "What would you think if I were to bring home a pair of intact, under-socialized, inbred Tasmanian Devils?"

On day 14 came the first soft-pitch, "You know, it's a two-hour roundtrip just to get a gallon of milk. I'm not sure Rachel is gonna be able to find good homes for all these puppies."

I have had a Blue Heeler rise from the dead in the floorboards of my pickup truck, lunge for my jugular vein, schmear my windshield, and pee down the defroster duct. I have attempted to fish a bottle of 50% dextrose, a simplex tube and a 14 gauge needle from my vet box without breaking eye contact and a hard body angle with a neutered male Australian Shepherd. Lessons learned from Mittsy, our staff behaviorist, have been found to be universal truths. Never risk removing a puppy from its mother or littermates prior to 6 weeks of age. Separation anxiety can be profound and difficult to manage.

"Your smile is like a breath of spring, your voice is soft as summer rain."

"What would you think about me bringing one home?"

Even with a career's worth of experience, being continually educated by a certified behaviorist, and flashing lights and warning signs galore, there would be only one answer. Still, I had to put up a bit of a fight. Hopefully, when she shredded the couch and the cleaning lady in the same day, I could get a thread of cred by not saying, "I told you so."

"You know Sheila, according to the Department of Agriculture, Tasmanian Devils entering Wisconsin from Wyoming, by way of Nebraska, require a six month quarantine," I pleaded.

Recalling the clairvoyance thing, Sheila had bought a soft-sided crate and notified the airline. The puppy/Tasmanian devil, "Token." had spent the 14-hour cowboy work days with her littermates. At night, the displaced herd dog clung to Sheila's shoulder and slept. Black, tan and brindle, her little nose parted Sheila's auburn locks, as they flowed to the collar of her Carhartt.

It would have been downright hypocritical not to enroll Token in the Puppy Socialization classes that Mittsy taught at the Lake Mills Veterinary Clinic. Yet, I was in no hurry to be stripped of any assumed respect and be proven the laughingstock by my classmates who were also clients. Had it not been for Wisconsin's "no child left behind," and a teacher with an open-door policy for after-hours tutoring, we may have never escaped kindergarten.

The early days she was prone to spontaneously breaking into piranha mode. On two separate occasions, I excused myself during the ten o'clock news. When I returned, Sheila asked where I had gone.

"To get a road atlas and fill up the truck." She was puzzled, but the only "out" I could imagine if the puppy launched into another spontaneous "Token Rage," was to load her up and drive her back to the ranch.

It has been said that a pet has a tendency to evolve into the likeness of her family. I had seen it a hundred times at the clinic. Joe and Laura Peterson were not done mourning the loss of their

 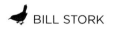

beloved Jasmine the day they brought Ava home. Fully realizing there would never be another Jas, they looked forward to a puppy new and wonderful. The next frame is of Joe and Laura standing in the lobby. As 4-month-old Ava scrambled innocently for the treats Mittsy had scattered on the floor, they stood slack-jawed and tattered. Their jeans and Packer hoodies looked as if they had sleep-walked into a lion's den wearing road-kill flavored BVDs.

Normally a jovial couple, we stifled the laughter and pulled out our best "leash walk and Kong" line of advice, and assured them that calm people have calm pets. A seasoned officer of the law, Joe reminded me that he was licensed to carry a sidearm and was not opposed to using it. Standing squarely in a position of believing my own B.S., I was not so convinced.

Somehow, not unlike a kid with colic, those days seemed to quickly fade. By virtue of Sheila's grace, Mittsy's expertise and in spite of me, she has settled into a solid companion. She will win every round of "rabbit carcass" hide and go seek, but has taken to trotting next to the horses, rather than trying to heel them.

I can scientifically explain her tendency to tree every rodent on our 6.8 acres. I share her concern over fireworks, gunshots and my son. Her obligatory and obnoxious manner of introducing herself to other dogs, and her fear of a day-old barn swallow I could expound upon for minutes.

What I have yet to pin an evolutionary or survival mechanism on is the threat posed by airborne snow. Put yourself in proximity of a shovel, broom or bucket tractor capable of elevating a measure of snow, and you have yourself a snarling, growling 44 lb ball of herd-dog terror.

On an evening early in the epic winter of 2010, I set out to clear the drive of the six or so inches of good ball-making snow. On cue, Token crouched and growled, waiting for her first victim. Standardly, my shoveling pattern revolves around preservation of my lumbar vertebrae. I will work from the center, pushing the snow as long as it will. Eventually it'll curl over the top of the shovel and have to be thrown to the curb. Alternating between pushing and throwing, the pup and my spine get a bit of half-time.

For the sake of variety, and curious, I decided to see how long she could go. Gathering my breath and ready to start, she squinted her left eye and slow nodded, "Give it a try, old bald guy."

We went up the drive and over the fence. We came back down and under. Still going strong, neither of us would show weakness. The higher I threw, the more times she would shred it — leaping and gnashing — before it settled to earth.

By the time we got from the garage to the barn, around the monument oak and back, the shovel count was at 150. Her genetic tenacity and stubbornness by association with her mom was impressive. As I shoveled, I thought. Years previous I had a Frisbee-playing Labrador named Cooder. I recalled the day I had to say goodbye. His hips would no longer lift him off the ground.

As the war raged on, I knew I could never deal with the notion I had hastened the demise of Token's hips for even a day. In her best interest and love of her mother, I laid the shovel at her feet.

At which, she promptly launched into the night to rearrange the goats.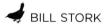

BILL STORK

The Rock

One of my favorite projects is building rock walls. I lack the good sense or patience to use small rocks that are easy to handle. Each occupies a large space in a wall, but takes some combination of brute strength, engineering, and colorful commentary to position. After the glaciers deposited them randomly across Wisconsin, farmers for centuries have piled rocks in fence lines and ditch banks so they could plow without breaking equipment.

My masterpiece started with three stones that were conservatively a half-ton each, on the far corner of the house. The stones were progressively smaller as the gradient rose, and ended at the front door. Mom had recently been diagnosed with Parkinson's disease. A wonderful woman, she had never been particularly agile. Now she would need sure footing when she came to visit her grandkids. I was figuratively and literally one rock short of a load. It had to be large, with a flat texture for traction and no divots that could pool water and freeze.

Southern Wisconsin has no shortage of rocks, but timing was crucial. By mid-May, wildflowers and weeds overtake ditches and fence lines, making finding and extraction a challenge. Within earshot of I-94 and just west of Lake Mills is Airport Road. There's no airport, but it does have beautiful rolling hills and plenty of rocks. It is there, by pure chance and dumb luck, we found our honey. Most things don't hold up to closer inspection, but this one was even better. Having spied it standing in the corner of a field, it was the perfect dimension, shape and texture.

There was no hiding the purpose in my approach. The farmer shifted his weight and looked at his boots. When he looked up, he held onto an "I suppose," and asked if we needed help with loading. That was our specialty, so I respectfully declined. An hour later, I backed the John Deere trailer square to the big flat rock. My son Calvin hand signaled as the 2" oak ramps ended at the edge of the rock. We cradled it in a tow strap, hooked up to the cable winch

Fifteen minutes later, my 50-pound kindergartner was feeling like King Kong, having learned his first lesson in physics after pulling the 300-pound rock all by himself. Dad was trembling with excitement.

A few months later, I was treating a sick calf on the very same farm. I once again thanked the farmer, describing how perfectly the stone served its purpose. Only then did he mention it had been the cornerstone and marker for that field.

In 2012, tractors turn 500 horsepower and seed is placed precisely by global positioning and soil maps. Not on the Kassube farm. For 100 years, and to this day, 25-horse, 2-cylinder museum pieces pull two bottom plows. Seed is placed by intuition and the accumulated experience of three generations. The rows were always as straight as the hood ornament on the 70-year-old tractor, lined up on a 3x2ft piece of granite that is now a stepping stone on Elm Point Road.

A gentleman is at least as likely to wear OshKosh B'gosh bib overalls as a tuxedo and black tie. And the greatest acts of generosity don't involve the exchange of a single dime. ⬡

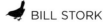 BILL STORK

The Cat Dancer

I remember clearly driving west on Dodge County Highway 19 early in the fall of 2008, and listening in horror as the stock market crashed. To say the past few years have been a challenge would be an understatement and an insult to those who have struggled. But it's not our first recession.

The last five years have drawn comparison to the mid-eighties; years I spent in high school and college. Though I remember the headlines in the newspaper, I never went without, largely thanks to a union heavy equipment operator at the top of his trade, and a mother who lived frugally and wasted nothing. Though Dad never missed an opportunity to provide for his family, he never missed an opportunity to be with us.

When we were together June through August, there is a pretty good chance you would find us near water — fishin' or swimming in it; water skiing on top of it. Our tow-boat was a 19-foot aluminum V-hull inboard/outboard. Next to the ski-hook was a cute little cartoon drawing of a Native American girl. Her eyes were originally black, but in a failed attempt to impress a young lady, I daubed them blue. Across the stern, bold and capitalized, was "CAT DANCER."

The Cat Dancer would never be mistaken for a tournament ski boat. Slightly more agile than a tug boat, she was pushed around by a 4-cylinder Chevy with a slightly noisy lifter in the third cylinder.

This feature was not lost on the Amazing Dick Bass. He was known to use the polite "tick tick" as a metronome. He would sit in the rear seat and play banjo in time with the motor as we would water ski.

She hauled and pulled our family and friends around the lakes of central Illinois for a decade and a half. By the time I made it to the University of Illinois, she became the perfect escape for land-locked students in Champaign-Urbana for summer sessions of pure intellectual enlightenment.

Mysteriously, the Cat Dancer reliably developed a seasonal mechanical failure that always seemed to resolve shortly after final exams were turned in. No technician or father was able to explain how she could run so well all summer, and develop the same malfunction each fall, shortly before mid-terms.

She served us well through four years of veterinary school. By the time I took the oath to serve and protect the human-animal bond on May 15th, 2002, the Cat Dancer was spent. With nothing that resembled trade value, she was recycled like an empty can of Budweiser. (Recall, this story is set in central Illinois.)

Upon graduation, I left the Land of Lincoln. Shortly after migrating across the Cheddar Curtain, I had a business and a piece of property. Back home, Dad had an 18-foot tandem axle Holsclaw trailer and no boat. Raised by recession-era parents and armed with a cutting torch and a welder, in short order we had a 16-foot work trailer. A construction worker with 40 years of experience and a scrap pile full of angle iron, it was not about to be overloaded or break down. Which is not to say I didn't try.

My mom meticulously (a polite way of saying she nearly drove my dad nuts) primed and painted the removable sideboards John Deere Green. Not to claim superiority over orange or red tractors, but to pay homage to the Johnny Popper: the tractors that planted 40 acres of Macon County, Illinois in popcorn in 1941, saving our family farm from the Great Depression. Dad's first job as a mechanic was working in a John Deere dealership, delivering and fixing the 2-cylinder work horses.

The trailer was used to haul everything from two tons of clay and a gas kiln, to dressers and mattresses every time a friend would separate from, or reconcile with, their mates. Dad left the bow winch on the tongue, so I could drag huge wheels of oak up the ramps intact, and then take them home to split them with the predecessor to the monster maul. Dad fashioned an old blacksmith's tool and a splitting wedge into a tool that could barely be lifted.

Not that we needed the wood to heat the house, but it was better than therapy and safer than alcohol. ❧

 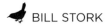 BILL STORK

Keep Your Eye on the Ball

In a recent appearance at the Stoughton Opera House, Michael Perry opened by thanking the standing room only audience:

"You have just braved a full-on blizzard and paid twenty dollars to see a 47-year-old man in work boots and Levis stand on stage and tell stories, who knows absolutely nothing. He knows this to be fact, because he has a 13-year-old daughter to remind him daily."

Amen, brother Mike. Being a man of science (and feeling a bit feeble), I conducted a formal study, over a mug of Rocky's Revenge at the Tyranena Brewing Company. As the research reveals, Parental Retardation appears to be a nearly universal affliction among folks who have managed to sire or birth children who eventually and inevitably go on to become teenagers.

Undaunted and oblivious, we parents search for, and hope to optimize, those "teachable moments." Last Saturday night on our way home from his last day in the terrain park at Alpine Valley, my 15-year-old son served one up like a fast ball right over a silver platter.

After 12 years of hockey and in need of a spring sport, he has decided to try baseball. I first confirmed that he was aware it is frowned upon to lower your shoulder and check the first baseman into right field as you round the bag and head for second. "Yeah, but what about charging the catcher?" he asked. "You have to get there first," I reminded him.

Fully aware of the inarguable truths established in paragraph one, I had his attention. In the sense that he was trapped in the passenger seat and had exhausted the battery on his phone posting video of his 540s on Instagram. There is always the risk that if I pass the opportunity I may not get it back. Not to mention, at home with space to demonstrate I could easily lose my cred. I couldn't hit my butt with both hands and a kindergartner could kick a beach ball past me in a headwind, but I know Kishan Khemani* and I can talk the talk. Mindful of the reason Chuck Berry never wrote a song more than 2 minutes long, I commenced hardcore parenting.

"Calvin, baseball is a game of awareness and preparedness. Always show up in a clean uniform, jersey tucked and hat on straight. On defense, know what you're gonna do with the ball, before it is pitched. Know how many outs there are, what the count is, and who the batter is on deck. Watch the batter's stance and body language to anticipate where he wants to hit the ball. When the pitcher goes into his windup, always be on your toes. Hands off your knees, butt down and head up. You make a catch with your whole body. Never reach when you can get in front of the ball. Face the play and move sideways when you can. And never forget the second commandment of baseball, **Use Two Hands.**"

Soccer may be the "Beautiful Game," and horse racing the "Sport of Kings," but baseball is much more than "America's Pastime." It has been called sport's greatest metaphor for life. The first commandment of baseball is "Keep your eye on the ball." We shout it through cupped hands at little leaguers and in stadiums at multi-cajillion dollar professionals. Yet we would be well served to stop... and think.

While one of, if not the most often uttered clichés in all of sports, "keep your eye on the ball." is also one of the most penetrating and universally applicable truths.

Hypothetically speaking, you may find yourself applying for admission to the University of Illinois College of Veterinary Medicine. Competing for one of 80 spots, against 900 applicants, all of whom are at least as qualified as you. As you greet and shake the hands with the admissions committee, you notice that the chair of the physiology department has particularly thick calluses, the cardiologist sports an Ohio State lapel pin, and the theriogenologist is wearing a distinctive pair of Luchese cowboy boots. Whether weaving into conversation your father who worked construction all his life, that Woody Hayes is just short of a deity, and your friend Carl Eads, the national champion team roper, had any influence on your eventual admission is the stuff of pure speculation.

As professionals, the difference between survival and success can be keeping your eye on the ball. For Erich Wollin, it may be recognizing that Effie is usually the third cow on the west side of the

 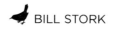 BILL STORK

parlor, but today she was last in her group. For Jed Hirschi riding 90,000 acres of Wyoming, it means that one of your 1500 Angus cows is bawling; her calf is sick and not nursing, and she is uncomfortable. At the Lake Mills Veterinary Clinic, our receptionist Claire notices that Bindy stops to urinate twice from the car to the building, suggesting that her 5 lb weight loss could be a consequence of diabetes or renal insufficiency.

My dad ran construction cranes capable of placing 500 tons of steel through a keyhole 250 feet away. In 45 years on the levers and clutch, no one ever got hurt and no metal bent. He showed up for work each day well-rested, well-fed and prepared. He wouldn't lift a cinder block with a cherry picker until the machine had been oiled, greased and inspected. If he or his iron workers were getting tired or the winds too strong, the load would be rigged and leveled. He gathered the men and informed them in language colorful and unique to the construction trade, yet inappropriate for a family publication, they would show up the next day rested and clear of mind.

Whether parents, partners, friends or those who serve, by living aware we can start to more completely fulfill our potential on this planet. The 5th grade teacher who notices that a student has worn the same clothes for three days straight, or does not have a coat and gloves for recess. Mail carriers who recognize when an elderly resident has not collected the mail. We may see that a friend simply does not take his usual place in conversation. We can notice the difference between polite and depressed, paralyzed and unable to step forward and ask for help.

We have come to live as slaves to our agendas, with urgencies both real and perceived. Let us downshift and ditch the blinders. Once we've recognized a friend in need, let us take our hands from our knees and our eyes off the computer screen. Help can be as simple as a word, a hand, or an ear to someone who is down.

Those 10 minutes are, without doubt, more valuable than the first two contestants on "Idol." ❧

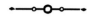

*Kishan Khemani is one of my best friends and student of all that is beautiful as it relates to the game of baseball. When he played high school baseball, his coach would throw all the gloves in a barrel, excepting the catcher. For the first two weeks of practice they used a piece of plywood with a strap on the back, instead of the glove. You will never see Kish catch a ball without using both hands. St. Louis Cardinals third baseman David Freese very nearly lost the World Series by letting a routine fly ball career off the heel of his glove.

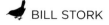

Mule Skinner Blues

We would never think to call any song with a guitar, bass and drums, "Beatles Music." It would be equally absurd to refer to every symphony as "Beethoven Music." However, put five musicians on stand-up bass, banjo, fiddle, mandolin and guitar around one microphone, singing perfect pitch harmonies high and lonesome, and it is Bluegrass Music.

The players will be well-dressed, punctual and polite, all the while singing of desperation, drinking, and drought, or about God. It is so because collectively Lester Flatt, Earl Scruggs, Chubby Wise and Howard Watts, along with Bill Monroe, were The Original Bluegrass Boys. It is Bill Monroe who dictated what Bluegrass Music would be, and specifically what it would not.

Born in 1911 to a family of fiddlers and guitar players, Bill was relegated to the mandolin — the least desirable instrument. He was asked to remove half the strings, so as to "not make so much noise." Yet in the nearly 60 years of performing and recording to follow, he would make the instrument his own and define a genre; one that has survived intact and still growing today. Posthumously and kindly referred to as enigmatic, Mr. Monroe spoke very little, to very few, offstage. The complexity and prolificacy of his music could not belie the genius within.

One of the few to whom Bill opened up, and a master in his own right, Peter Rowan was an early protégé and a latter day Blue Grass Boy. He asked Bill how he could play "Mule Skinner Blues" 250 times a year.

"You don't," was his response.

After a pause, and satisfied with the depth and duration of the crease in the young guitar player's brow he explained, "Peter, you don't play the song, you further the music. Every time out, every man up, you look for a note, a word, a phrase that you can play or sing better than or differently than the night before. In doing so, you never play the same song twice, and the music is always alive."

William Smith Monroe is the indisputable Father of Bluegrass Music, but he's got nothing on William Ernest Stork. My dad was a heavy equipment operator. Not one of his inventions would ever bear a patent, but were born of necessity and fully functional. His body of work includes everything from libraries, gymnasiums and bridges to a nuclear power plant.

Every day on the job he showed up thirty minutes early, equipped and informed. When the workday was done, and he rested on his tailgate, there was a little more completed than what was expected.

"Keep the boss man eating steak and he will keep you eating hamburger; when the boss man goes to eating hamburger, you go hungry..." we heard once or twice (a day).

"Son, it don't matter if you're loadin' dirt on a dump truck or settin' fuel rods, do it a little smoother, quicker and cleaner than last time."

At his retirement party, Dad introduced me to a circle of operators and iron workers. They joked at how Dad would use the first 15 minutes of lunch break to eat the sandwich Mom had packed, and the second half to rest. It could be the seat of a Cat D-12 with his feet on the dash, or on the tracks of a 500 ton Manitowoc tower rig, but you could hear "Red" snoring over a jackhammer.

When he walked away, they turned serious. "I tell you what about your dad, the boss man would tell him what to do, and you knew in his eyes he had a better way, but he'd climb on the crane and do things just exactly like he was told."

"If it wasn't obvious, he'd make sure the boss could see the wheels were about to fall off. He'd dog off the machine and crawl down the tracks. 'You know, I was just thinkin' about how we...', he'd start with the boss man, who was standing heels and elbows tight, with the brim of his hard hat low and chin buried between his thumb and index finger. Feeling his fat being pulled from the fryer, you'd see his shoulders drop, 'Oh, yeah, that's a real good idea...'"

"From that day forward, the boss man would just show your dad the blueprints and point at a pile of steel."

After four decades on the job, when Dad finally hung up his hard

BILL STORK

hat, he did it with the respect of everyone he had ever worked with.

He is a self-proclaimed, "dumb old construction worker," yet rest assured that every weld, I-beam, brick and bolt still stands true some 50 years later. Thanks to 40 years of hard work, good health and the unconditional support and frugality of my mom, he retired with a good living. That said, Heavy Equipment Operator (and lifetime member of IUOE) only starts to define who he is.

On April 9, 1956 in St. Patrick's Catholic Church, he married Alma Ann Beasley. Before friends, family and God, he swore to love her richer and poor, in sickness and health, until death do they part. That is exactly what he did.

On March 3, 1965, I was born. From the first day I could remember, there would be nary a doubt that Mom and I were his first and only priority.

There could have been 35 taverns and two strip joints between the Clinton Nuclear Power Plant and 1195 Nickey Avenue, but if Dad was not at the dinner table, we knew exactly where he was. He worked tirelessly to provide for his family, yet if I were to receive an award for perfect attendance in 8th grade, or play a solo in the Jazz band, he never missed. If I needed someone to throw grounders or weld my mower, he was never too tired.

As parents, we sit on the sidelines and in the bleachers so we can share the joy of success, absorb some of the pain, and lend perspective to inevitable defeat. In doing so, we hope there is a thread of credibility when a kid might need a nudge in a different direction. (Dad called it a size 9-1/2 Red Wing in the butt.)

Father's Day is near. If we are so fortunate, our kids will make us cards and buy us books, fishing rods, grills and house slippers. Let's take the day to not only appreciate, but to ensure we are the examples they deserve.

As my father before me, help us build relationships and legacy from which our children can grow. At 16, I could recite every one of his sayings and sound bites, line and verse; yet it is actions that define my dad. At 48, with two kids of my own, I can only hope to live up to them. ❧

The Wave

By 1982 my dream of becoming a veterinarian was in overdrive. A misnomer, there was not so much as a pond in sight from Lakeview High School. However, it was but 250 yards from the Brush College Animal Hospital, which in turn was 4-1/2 blocks from home.

So, like Billy from Family Circus, several days a week and every weekend I would go from home to the clinic, to school and back to the clinic. There Dr. William Van Alstine graciously provided every opportunity to be involved in the intricacies of companion animal medicine and practice ownership, and $2.85 an hour. If on any entrance exam or interview I were to be grilled on cage cleaning, baseboard scrubbing, mopping, defecation decontamination, weed pulling or kennel painting, I knew it cold.

Woefully deficient was my exposure to production animal medicine. So when spring break rolled around in my junior year of high school, I contemplated beach or mountains. Looking to beef up my resume, I opted for a week on "the farm."

From the road, "the farm" looked like Sanford and Son meets House on the Rock. Had American Pickers been on the air 30 years ago, they would have never left McLean County, Illinois. Butch and Nancy were lifelong friends of our family and were more than happy for me to move in.

The educational value of the trip will forever be in debate, and I am still trying to bring my cholesterol in line.

Like the 9ft tall, ill-mannered grizzly from Jimmy Buffet's epic "God's Own Drunk." Butch wore a naked upper lip above a full red beard that, in the absence of a neck, merged with or substituted for chest hair. He wore his blue chambray work shirt (yes, singular) unbuttoned most of the year; Butch was well insulated by 10 years of Nancy's cooking. His head was the size and shape of BJ Raji's football helmet, with a laugh to match. Mostly at his own jokes which, after a several trips to confession, and Father Walton's sug-

 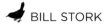 BILL STORK

gestion of a half dozen Our Fathers and Hail Marys, have left no permanent scar.

There's an old joke. A Texas rancher drawls, "I get up every morning, git in my pickup truck, and drive. By sunset, I git to the other side of my ranch." Guy from Wisconsin, "Yup, I had a truck like that." Butch bought it. It was a 1970 Chevy half-ton; the kind with green on the top, white down the middle, and rust on the bottom. Four mismatched bald tires that I would not trust on an empty hay rack completed the ensemble.

With Butch on the driver side for 10 years, she was darn near at capacity, and if you put a bowling ball on the passenger seat, it would have rolled through the driver's door. There is no doubt you could have taken the shocks and springs off the passenger side, boxed 'em up, and sold them as new. Rather than "three on the tree," there was scrap iron through the floorboard. An old mud flap, four rivets, and natural ventilation kept most of the exhaust out as muffler and tailpipe were long gone. With the clutch of little value, mostly it was "find and grind."

From thirty yards and a rearview, you couldn't tell Nancy from Butch. Enterprising beef farmers as they were, they looked for a niche market. Touting cholesterol levels less than tofu, they bought a handful of 8-week-old Texas Longhorn calves, and pastured them in broken-down fences that would not contain a 20-year-old returned Jersey fair calf.

In two years and a half dozen neighborhood round-ups, they were ready to go to market. Opting to take their product straight to the people, they set up near the meat case at the local Piggly Wiggly. Grass-fed and grassroots, acting as their own spokesmodels. It is a mystery to this day why sales were perpetually slow.

The accommodations and transportation may not have been plush, but the education was priceless. Being the youngest and the dumbest, I was designated to pull newborn calves onto the hood of a 1950 Plymouth, turned upside down and hitched behind a tractor. Mom would follow into a maternity pen so the calf could be licked and nursed in privacy.

I learned about setting corner posts, cross braces, and splicing woven wire. I will not soon forget which pocket not to put pliers in, so as to not get knocked down by an old Hereford cross named "Red" scratching her head. Always applicable, I mastered how to walk across a cow yard without your boots being pulled off your feet.

Early on, I perfected the art of going to town for coffee, lunch and parts. Butch greeted every familiar car and truck, which was most, with a wave. His cavernous cranium never deviating, his free right hand would trace the shape of, and a few inches above, the steering wheel and dashboard. As he neared his reach and the center of the truck, he'd rotate his palm uphill toward the passenger door as the car passed.

All the above being the absolute truth, one week in Farmer City, Illinois, 30 years ago, left an indelible impression on this city boy. With living in a small town comes opportunity. Maybe not unique, but more accessible, is familiarity and interdependence. If we let it, we can appreciate and respect folks at a deeper and more significant level when they are one of a few, rather than a blur on the tollway. ❧

 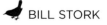 BILL STORK

Uncle Con

Early April 1936, well before first light, Frank sat motionless in thought. A shadow on the dusty floor from a single naked bulb, enveloped by last Sunday's fried chicken, this morning's coffee and 70-year-old pine, he thumbed the strap of his OshKosh overalls. His left hand surrounded a white diner coffee mug like a shot glass, long since cold, but well before the answers would come. The chair creaked and lid rattled as he dragged the handle of the granite coffee boiler across the wood stove.

Two hundred miles to the north, in Chicago — like every city — The Great Depression had gutted the land. One in four men was without work; the fortunate fought for survival. In the Heartland, grain prices had fallen to $0.13 per bushel. At 30 bushels per acre, an 80-acre farm could earn less than $250 per year, a fraction of what would make a farm payment. Many burned corn for heat; it was cheaper than coal.

Soon after sunrise, yet far from earshot, like John Henry in West Virginia, a chain gang would commence. The rhythmic "grunt, ping, thud" of steel driving spikes into railroad ties would continue 'til sunset, bringing the Norfolk and Southern Railroad north, and bisecting three acres from the farm.

By first frost the steel rails would carry three cars of popcorn 100 miles south to St. Louis. Two rows at a time behind a John Deere B, Frank had planted every tillable inch of Christian County clay that he had a claim to, bringing to fruition a plan and a prayer made somewhere during the second cup of coffee, and closed on a handshake. A man in St. Louis owned movie houses. Folks lived for simple pleasures; when they could scrape together a few nickels and a dime, they would treat the family to a show and a snack.

Born in 1866, Frank would see the farm through the forties as WWII united the country. He and wife Agnes would have seven children, all of whom would move away, excepting Conrad, who never left the farm, and never married.

His nephew Bill wasn't born on the farm, but you couldn't keep him off it. As a boy, Bill would practice welding pieces of scrap steel gathered by Con. When he was old enough to reach the clutch, (and anytime school, the Chrysler garage, or the U.S. Navy would spare him), he could be found on the farm, riding a Putt-Putt Johnny, planting, plowing or picking.

Bill had the heart of a farmer but not the stomach. When he returned from four years in the Seabees, he entered the apprenticeship for the Operating Engineers and became a heavy equipment operator and mechanic.

This is my family farm. Frank was my great-grandfather; Conrad, my namesake uncle. Bill, of course, is my Dad.

Memories of Uncle Con's farm are defining: family reunions, driving lawn mowers, hunting among the stubble for corn dropped by the combine, and pressing apples from the orchard. The John Deere cap on my head isn't because it matches my coveralls. If it was green and made in Moline, Uncle Con would have one and a spare. It was there I drove my first tractor: a John Deere 4020, 100 horsepower, made the year I was born.

My most vivid memory of the farm is sweet corn. Around 4:30 in the evening, the third week of July — give or take — the phone would ring:

"This is Con, you better come and get your corn before the 'coons do."

He would plant five acres of sweet corn for family, and folks in town. We would load friends and cousins in the back of dad's yellow '68 Chevy, and hightail it 25 miles south on Illinois Route 48. When we got to the farm, Dad would drop the tailgate and back through the field. The kids would pick and toss ears of "Garwood Supreme," until the 396 was growling and corn was rolling off the side walls. Back in town when the neighbors saw the Chevy heavy half, bumper- draggin' down Nickey Avenue, they'd come quick with brown paper bags.

 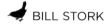 BILL STORK

Ask anyone who lived through the Depression: they will speak of what they had, not what they didn't. Nothing, not a kernel of corn, was wasted. The next days would be spent boiling, carving, cleaning and canning corn, until all that was left was a mountain of naked cobs, from which we made jelly.

Uncle Con farmed through the '60s, knowing he would be the last generation of Storks on the family farm. Raw-boned and strong as a spool of number 9 wire, wearing the family uniform — OshKosh bib overalls — he sat at the same kitchen table his father had 40 years previous, lost in his own thoughts. Tough as the soles of his boots, yet he was no match for the tumors that ravaged his pancreas. Cancer had taken his strength and reserves, but his senses were well intact.

Decisions made.

The next morning, the driveway would look like a Labor Day Parade: on rolled a roofer, insulator, electrician, plumber, an HVAC panel truck, and a crew of carpenters. By the time the ambulance would take him to St. Mary's hospital to numb the pain of his last few days, the old farm house stood proud as the day it was built. The shop was rewired and plumbed and the walls insulated and heated.

His sister, my aunt called in a fit. "Damned old fool is dying, and he just had the whole farm rebuilt." Dad smiled and nodded; he knew exactly what was on the old farmer's mind.

Six hundred and forty acres to the south was Bollinger Farms. As an upstart young farmer in the late '50s and '60s, Uncle Con was there when Tom Bollinger was short a wagon, or a tractor broke down. As time marched on and my uncle would be less able, Tom would return the gesture, as neighbors do.

By the time Uncle Con passed in 1975, son Steve Bollinger was looking to start a family of his own. Con's sisters came to claim plates, pictures, and mementos. Dad, his cousins and I divided welders, grinders and wrenches.

As far as Steve was concerned, born to farm in his father's footsteps, where better to start a life than a quarter mile from home in a brand-new, old, farmhouse.

Tractor-pulling fans will recognize "Money Pit" and "Top Gun." perennially in the NTPA top 10 machines in the Unlimited Division. Each tractor is equipped with three 12-Cylinder Allison Aircraft engines. Decommissioned from retired B-38 bombers from WWII, they were assembled in the shop Uncle Con had rebuilt, days before he died.

In the house lives Steve, his wife, and their children.

Not a soul named Stork has stuck a plow in the ground for over 40 years, but 50 years ago my uncle did a neighbor a good turn. Last Tuesday, my phone rang:

"Hey Bill, this is Steve Bollinger, y'all better come down and get your sweet corn." ◆

 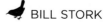

Hail the Workin' Man (and woman)

There were three deep potholes on East Grant Street. Monday through Friday, near 5 p.m., the overload springs on a 1975 3/4-ton Ford would slap, and the 460 would growl as Dad shifted down. Whether at 6 years old building an overpass in the sandbox with my Tonka articulating end loader and dump truck, or at age 16 blowing ulcers over pre-calculus, I was always in earshot. Like a victory lap, he'd idle past, swing wide, check both mirrors and back in.

If he parked under the basketball hoop, we were working on the neighbor's car after supper. In front of the kitchen, something was gonna get torched and welded. If he pulled in forward to the rear wheel wells, it was time to change the oil: every 1500 miles, recorded in magic marker between the 2x4's, just to the left of the vise from Uncle Con's farm.

In 30 minutes Mom, Dad, the neighbor with the exhaust leak, and I would be sitting down to supper at the three-leaf mahogany dinner table under a 12x36 oil reproduction of the Last Supper. It is only now, forty years on, that I can appreciate all I had to give thanks for when we bowed our heads and crossed our hearts.

In the 10 (or 16) hours since that pickup had rolled out the drive, somewhere in the 15 counties of central Illinois served by the International Union of Operating Engineers Local 965, there had been 125 pieces of steel set, 400 yards of concrete poured, and a mountain of fill dirt leveled. There was a Cat D10, crane, blade or picker that was hissing, cracking and cooling; backed in line, oiled, fueled and ready for tomorrow.

Sweaty, greasy, callused and tired was a crew of iron workers, pipe fitters, electricians and laborers heading to their families. Thanks to these men and women, there was a bridge, road, library, gymnasium, or power plant that was an honest day closer to the ribbon-cutting on the 10 o'clock news.

It was at that table over chicken fried steak and mashed potatoes that a hardcore respect for the "Working Man" was engraved on my soul, not by sermon but example. Today I speak "white coats and stethoscopes," but "Carhartts and Redwings" is my native tongue. For every bite of food, shred of common sense, and eight years of book learnin', I have to thank a construction worker, two millwrights, a machinist and carpenters, welders and pipe fitters — more than I can count.

The first Monday in September is Labor Day.

Somewhere amongst the parades and packing up the lake house, let's pause to dispense with the politics and celebrate and appreciate the men and women who work with their hands. Folks at the USPS like Linda and Dana who deliver Kohl's sale flyers and bank statements. Butch and Judy who haul 40,000 lbs of Crystal Farms cheese from Lake Mills, and bring us Vitamin C from San Diego all winter long.

Without Sterwald's to pull us out of ditches, Schuman's to keep rain off our head, John to keep the lights on, and Jensen's to keep clean water coming and dirty water away, we might be helpless.

So, next time you see a Hi-Vis vest and hard hat, make eye contact with a slow nod, a low wave and a wide berth. They'll know.

 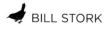 BILL STORK

Mrs. Haynes

Mrs. Haynes lived across Nickey Avenue from our family. I only knew her as a widow, smartly dressed and made up, whether she was mowing grass, shoveling snow, or going to the market. Wearing a clear plastic rain bonnet with blue trim hovering over a brand new perm and tied under her chin, she may have been five foot two, in perpetual motion dawn to dusk.

From her mailbox, four concrete steps led to the front door between two huge red potted geraniums. To one side of the porch, a two-seat white swing swayed lazily in the breeze, hidden in the shade. Her driveway had more cracks than a Kansas wheat field in the dust bowl. From the road, it descended to the left of the Japanese yew and wrapped the back side of the little red brick home, forming a parking pad just off the garage and kitchen. Her ¾ acre lot more resembled a motocross course, with crab grass and a big black walnut tree by the front ditch. Her back lot line was marked by the stump of a long-dead oak that also served as second base in the empty lot where my friends and I played ball.

Summer mornings, the sun's rays would warm the heavy dew clinging to the tall grass of the infield of our neighborhood "field of dreams," forming a thin ground fog, and warming the 4x4 picture window through which Mrs. Haynes watched the world.

Through that window was her kitchen, where she seemed to live. Four oak arm chairs with pads tied through the spindles were neatly pushed under a small round kitchen table. The top was covered with the requisite plastic table cloth and last year's copies of "Better Homes and Gardens," recipe pages dog-eared and coupons clipped. An upright piano was pressed against the stairwell. Just past were two easels, from which every friend or family member had a meticulously brushed red hip-roof barn with silhouettes of horses and white fence, or sawmill and paddle wheel hanging in their kitchen or hallway. Two parakeets whistled and cackled, their cage doors always propped open.

Folks born near the turn of the century had gutted out The Great Depression and a world war. When they asked for "a little help," you didn't question their need. Mrs. Haynes called my mom: her mower wouldn't start. Could little Bill come and take a look?

At twelve, just old enough to feel a little swell in my chest, but no more a mechanic than I am today, I stuffed my pockets with the few tools I knew how to use, and a couple that looked manly. Brow creased, I angled across our yard and hers. With an 11/16 deep well socket, a farmer's match and four hard pulls, the 21" Crafts-man staggered to life. As the smoke cleared, I offered to take a few rounds, "just to make sure it was gonna stay runnin'."

Having learned a thing or two about selective hearing from Dad, I pretended not to notice when she tried to take over. My attempts to refuse payment proved futile and I just kept mowing, shoveling, picking up walnuts, and raking leaves, until I graduated from high school. She paid $7.50 for mowing and raking, $5.00 for shoveling (the walnuts I picked for free, but resold to my grandpa). Fair pay for the day, and plenty for Big Macs, malts and boat gas, with some left for saving.

In retrospect I would have done it all, plus clean her gutters, the parakeets' cages and fetched the newspaper... for a single slice of her cinnamon bread.

KFC vents their fryers over the entrance to the restaurant, satu-rating the parking lot with essence of "Original Recipe." Colonel Sanders had nothing on Mrs. Haynes. By the time Mom would poke her head around and call, "Mrs. Haynes has cinnamon bread!" I would be airborne. The sweet aroma had already wafted through her kitchen window and across the road. Absorbed in long division or sentence diagramming, I would sit bolt upright and fly over the first four steps from my bedroom to the landing of the stairs with a 150 lb THUD!

I'd cover the 100 yards from our door to hers as fast as my high-top Converse would carry me, trying to settle my breath in time to be polite. Attempts to make conversation were transparent at best: "Hi, Mrs. Haynes, how are, um...?"

"Oh you're right on time, I just pulled a loaf out of the oven," she would giggle modestly.

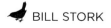

Wrapped intricately in two pieces of tin foil, cradled perfectly between my fingertips and elbow, I carried it sacred as a game ball in the Super Bowl. Carefully, Mom would lift the dome on the holy loaf. The crust was brown as a buckskin horse and flakey as a used car salesman. Perfect as a pebble in a pond, each concentric ring was butter-brushed and sprinkled evenly with cinnamon sweetness. Like the last tug on the straw before the malt goes *slurp!*, the gooey center begged for just one more swallow of milk.

Mrs. Haynes was my earliest recollection of the devastating effects of Alzheimer's disease.

The first sign of decline could have been the bread: a bit overdone, maybe a little chewy. In my earliest confirmation of the beholder and beauty, it was always perfect. When Mrs. Haynes, by definition proud and proper, was seen fetching the morning paper in her undergarments, and the mail in her nightclothes, there was no denial.

On Sunday, September 15, at 10:00 a.m., our family participated in the Walk to End Alzheimer's, in memory of Mrs. Virginia Haynes, Alma Ann Stork, Estol Beasley, and in support of tens of families we know personally and thousands worldwide devastated by this dehumanizing monster.

My daughter, Paige, rallied our family: "Everyone who ever knew my Grandma said she was the kindest person they had ever met. I believed them." she continued, "but when she was affected by Alzheimer's I was very young, and didn't really get to know her." "I don't want that to happen to families in the future." ❦

The Unstoppable Judy B

She could have been admitted through emergency at San Diego General. Dean Care would have covered her without question. Her niece, Hannah, would ensure she received the best of care, and her discomfort would never pass the little yellow face with the creased brow.

She could have caught a cab from Whiskey Pete's Truck Stop to Mountain View Medical Center in Las Vegas.

She could have rolled straight through security and onto the first class seat her daughter had booked out of Salt Lake City International.

But there were 40,000 pounds of fruit behind an '02 Peterbilt. Woodman's expected delivery by Friday noon, and it wasn't going to drive itself home. Her husband, Butch, had been truckin' for 38 years, but there wasn't enough caffeine in California to keep his eyes open another mile.

1,400 miles and 20 hours from home, the Jake brake growled full-throat as the 53-foot reefer leaned gently onto the shoulder of I-80 eastbound.

Knowing he may as well be talking to President Lincoln, "Judy, give me 150 miles and I'll be back at it," Butch croaked as he crawled into the sleeper.

The next thing he'd see that didn't look like the backside of his eyelids would be the "Come Again" sign, as she put Cheyenne in their rearview, 489 miles later, bound for Omaha.

Half a continent later, and nearly two days after her first attack, they'd dock the produce at Sun Prairie Woodman's. An hour after that, she would be in room 402 at St. Mary's Hospital. A constant-rate infusion pump delivered intravenous fluids through a catheter in her right arm to correct her dehydration. Antibiotics and morphine were piggy-backed to fight the pain and infection. A CT scan found a raging case of diverticulitis. Surgery would be scheduled, but not until she was *stronger*.

 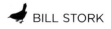 BILL STORK

Judy Barnes is just past 70 and 5'4." with her hair in curls. She walks softly, speaks softly and carries no stick. Yet, on the 120 acres near the intersection of County C and G known by one of the most cohesive families and inclusive circle of friends I have ever witnessed as "the farm"; if there is ever need for a final word, it will be hers.

Her left foot is as comfortable at the pedal of a Singer mending overalls as on the clutch of a Peterbilt hauling freight. No one has ever left her kitchen a stranger, or pushed back from her Christmas table empty-handed, heavy-hearted or hungry. At a time when compassion, common sense and accountability are endangered, look no further than her two sons and daughters.

Simply put, Judy B is a bastion of core values, strength and family. That being said, it is neither the topic of this piece, nor her identity.

For those who know her best, Judy's defining attribute is her gas.

Cleaning up after Thanksgiving dinner she can be simple, prolific and sustained. Marching through Kohls scouting pre-Christmas door-buster deals, in synchrony with every step she can be staccato and musical.

Andante or Allegro, Judy B is a virtuoso, having rendered flatulence a fine art.

Others, by virtue of genetics, medical conditions or PED's may come close, but it is in the presentation where Judy stands alone. Each movement is delivered humbly, and void of apology or bravado. The surgery would prove successful, but only after weeks of antibiotics and fluid diet. Judy lay in her hospital bed, surrounded by machines going "ping," fluid pumps, and family.

The surgeon, in a highly medical fashion, deadpanned, "The first step is for her to pass gas."

Her daughters and husband were precariously balanced between too stunned to speak and "be careful what you wish for." Like ducks in the desert, waiting and wishing for Judy to produce was uncharted waters.

It was in those waiting hours that I had opportunity to think.

From royalty to the rank and file, devout to agnostic, newborn to geriatric, not one of us is spared. Imagine, if you will, how history may have been altered by the mere fear of an uncontrolled expulsion. Let alone the physical act, how many first impressions have been flubbed with no second chance? We will never know the commencement addresses, sermons and speeches that may have inspired us to action, were it not for an orator's poor choice of side dishes and fear of a hypersensitive sound system.

By way of full disclosure, one too many clumps of cauliflower and a small animal veterinarian soon finds himself praying for three loud children and a cocker spaniel with an ear infection, or else he finds himself wishing for a creaking door through which to excuse himself to examine a slide under the microscope. Apropos, unless the patient is presented for a heart murmur or behavior problem.

The Krebs cycle is the bane of every college student, and the chemical pathway by which all fuel — from free-range bison burgers to fresh arugula — is converted to mechanical motion, meaningful thought and productivity. Methane is an obligate product of digestion.

Yet decorum dictates that, when faced with an excess, we refrain or apologize.

It is no less physiologic than a sneeze, yet when someone forcefully exhales, we say "Gesundheit," or "bless you." There was once a time when we thought a sneeze was an opportunity for evil spirits to enter the body. It seems abundantly clear how they escape.

So in honor of Judy, and for the better of us all, I propose that we simply and quietly decommission the fart. Place it alongside sneezing, coughing, snoring, and post-nasal drip. Not to be celebrated, or apologized; a privilege not to be abused. One can only dream of the efficiency and productivity to be gained the day when, once and for all, we no longer live in fear. ❧

 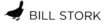 BILL STORK

Smokin' Weed

It was mid-July 2005. Recently removed from my home and half of all I had worked for, at times the only thing preventing me from dropping to the fetal position was the thought of having to stand up again. Buddhists tell us not to try and escape the low times, but to explore them. I was simply trying to survive.

Relegated to the ranks of a part-time dad, and trying to "redefine." I had taken up residence on the same five acres where Becky and Lyle Wallace had planned to raise their three boys, a couple horses, a few pigs, and some vegetables.

On the north side of the house was a perfect rocking chair porch that overlooked the monument maple, and a one-acre "Field of Dreams." Three mostly rotten, once white boards surrounded the paddock, clinging precariously to fence posts that stood at any angle from 90 to nearly 45 degrees. Remnants of insulators and broken strands of number 16 wire suggested that someone had once hoped to keep animals. A rusted red, twelve foot gate hung limp off a broken corner post, nary an angle brace to be found.

I stood on the concrete in my best pair of Levi's and three-year-old Red Wing 402's, contemplating how to get from where I was. The rising sun knifed the morning dew between the hip-roof dairy barn and wood shed. Steam rolled off the dark black brew in the bottom of the hand-thrown, wood-fired mug gifted by my friend, Mark the potter.

I imagined a soccer goal on each end of the pasture. The third fence post by the road would be the north sideline; a pair of sweatpants, the south. Some days we could pull three pieces of cardboard out of the recycling bin and play baseball. When Calvin could hit the ball into the weeds on the next farm, we could switch to whiffle ball.

Norman Rockwell and Kishan Khemani would be proud, but today there was a problem. As if Lyle and Becky had planted them, the entire field was covered with the most majestic stand of burdock this side of the redwood forests. Conceivable to anyone who knew Lyle, in the sense that burdock is used as an herb in Asian cooking, and its roots are coveted by homeopaths for their ability to "purify" the blood and support the liver. Most importantly, it sells for $14.95 per pound.

On this particular day my blood seemed fine, and liver in perfect working order. Bacon and eggs are more my style than pasture weeds on spinach, and it seemed there must be better ways to pull down $15.00.

After a couple sick cows and a full book of small animal appointments, I picked up my son and daughter in time for a late lunch. As I was picking up the dishes, my daughter moped into the kitchen, shoulders hanging low and on the brink of tears. She had been out exploring the property in her favorite hockey hoodie. "Chicks with Sticks" on the front, a silver star next to her name and jersey number on the back, it was now covered permanently with George de Mestral's inspiration for the creation of Velcro: burdock seeds.

To a dad in need of a physical outlet for his emotional pain, this meant war.

Man has been battling burdock for centuries. In a recent installment of his Sunday column, Michael Perry recounts a similar situation. His weapon of choice was a tractor and brush hog. Though I had no four foot, diesel-powered weapon of mass destruction, failure was not an option. Ace Hardware was only 20 minutes down Interstate 94. An hour later I returned, armed with a Stihl FS 90 commercial weed trimmer with brush blade, and two gallons of 25:1.

Lest another garment suffer the same fate as Paige's sweatshirt, I needed a uniform impenetrable to the noxious weed and its heinous seed pod. There simply was not time to consider afternoon temperatures approaching 80 degrees or the first impression of my new neighbors. I geared up. Like hiking to a down cow in a blizzard, I pulled out the rip-stop, 100% rubber, Helly Hansen foul weather fishing jacket and tugged the drawstring tight around my face and waist. With the pants to match pulled over my 5-buckle Lacrosse overshoes, I was bulletproof.

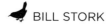 BILL STORK

With three pushes on the primer and one pull, the German machine growled to life. Outnumbered like Rambo, I waded into battle, vowing not to come out until every stalk was on the ground or I passed out from dehydration.

Three hours and two tanks of fuel later, I walked through the broken red gate, laid my weapon down, stripped off my armor, and poured the sweat from my boots. With a skid-loader and bale forks I plowed and stacked the carcasses into a compacted pile the size of a UPS truck. With one match, five gallons of Boy Scout water and a six pack of Rocky's Revenge, the first battle was won.

By midnight the flames died and the smoke from what had been a field of weed eighteen hours previous filtered through the maple branches. I am not sure whether there was any correlation, but I did develop a powerful case of the munchies. If I achieved higher thought or deeper state of awareness, I do not recall. What I do know is that, for that one day, I had a small victory.

The war would wage for months. By way of chemical warfare, a Ransome's 23 horse ZTR and a 10 Ton Bomag vibrating asphalt roller, the dream that started with a cup of coffee and a ruined hoodie would become a reality. ❧

Vet School

BILL STORK

I'm a Pepper

If I am able to continue to write, the papers willing to print, and you are kind enough to read these weekly ramblings, you will eventually become acquainted with The Amazing Dick Bass.

Hopefully you are already; if not by name, then by his spirit that lives in all who knew him.

The Amazing Dick Bass was a professor of electrical engineering at Georgia Tech, and on the forefront of alternatively powered vehicles. He played banjo, piano, guitar, and mandolin, and sang bluegrass and gospel music.

He served breakfast in homeless shelters and wired houses with Habitat for Humanity. ADB was one of the most understated and over-accomplished humans I've ever known. He was devoutly Christian in all his actions, and never judged or recruited.

Never has the phrase "let no man (or woman) die in vain" been more apropos. As the New Year nears and we pause for introspection, allow me to offer the defining trait of The Amazing Dick Bass as a possible resolution.

You don't need to know how to pick or grin, and you don't need to know a zener diode from a circuit. All you need is fifty cents a day (adjusted for inflation).

The trait that defined Dick Bass is one we can all emulate. Every sunrise, meal, walk, bike ride, breath, and certainly every person was special in some way.

His single-handed transformation of 4:00 p.m., Monday-Friday could be his defining achievement.

During pursuit of his Ph.D., exhausted and saddle sore (on a Tuesday afternoon), he suddenly realized he was a "Pepper." He asked the obvious question of his lab-mates.

Putting down their pocket protectors and idling their HPs, they moved toward the door. In formation they marched down the hall. The ranks swelled as their voices echoed off the marble floor, "I'm a Pepper, she's a Pepper, wouldn't you like to be a Pepper too!"

From that day forward, on cue from the Amazing Dick Bass, the entire Electrical Engineering department took a daily break from advancing science. They likely did not continue to chant the Dr. Pepper jingle, but they did look forward to connecting with those they might otherwise simply pass in the hallway.

I find it nearly impossible to get out of bed without something to look forward to. According to my banker, retirement will be near 125 years of age, and next summer's bike ride is too distant. Look for something, or somebody to enjoy each day. You may find yourself inspired and energized, and you will do the same for a friend.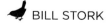

It Ain't Easy Bein' Green

The Cat Dancer sat idling, facing due east up the length of Eagle Creek. I stood on the bow, sifting grounds of campfire coffee through my teeth. Off the stern, the 65-foot tow rope meandered across the glass-calm surface of the lake. Gary the Hog Farmer checked the straps on his neoprene gloves and vest.

The Amazing Dick Bass sat next to the motor cover, looking like a wounded soldier from the Civil War, playing a Sears and Roebuck banjo from the same era. His head was wrapped in a shower cap and Ace bandage in order to keep 18 sutures dry (stitched by a second year veterinary student who will remain anonymous). The wound was carnage from a failed attempt at slalom skiing just before the sunset last. He loped through "When Johnny Comes Marching Home," the ticking of the 4-cylinder Chevy keeping time. Cooder, my 8-month-old yellow lab sat facing rearward, barely interested.

As the first rays of morning knifed the fog hanging low over Lake Shelbyville, the day began. I tossed the remains of the coffee, dropped the throttle, and Gary slowly rose out of the water. A hopeful family of buzzards patrolled the sky as Gary shredded the imaginary slalom course. Holding a straight line and looking forward, I could feel the underpowered tugboat as Gary heaved with every turn, his ski sizzling on hard edge as he crossed the wake.

Body motionless, hands flying, Dr. Bass scorched a sunrise rendition of "Foggy Mountain Breakdown," still keeping time with the noisy lifter on cylinder #3. Cooder napped.

And so began day two of "Weekend at the Lake." After three months of trying to earn enough to make a dent in student loans, before going back to the academic "rock pile" for another 52 weeks, we took 48 hours of R&R and pulled out all the stops.

The starting lineup featured Gary the Hog Farmer, because he could drive the boat, back the trailer and is simply one of the finest humans on Earth; The Amazing Dick Bass, Cooder, and Elizabeth Clyde.

Elizabeth loved to water ski, is terminally cute, and had a Louisiana accent that said "welcome home." Her degree in biology from LSU landed her in the University of Illinois College of Veterinary Medicine, Class of 1992, and made us classmates. Two years of cooking classes from Justin (red wine, white wine, fish don't know what color the wine is!) Wilson rendered us soulmates. We had a deal: if the boat moved, she was invited. If she was brewing etouffee, I was there with bowl and spoon.

I'm all but certain the Cajun spice fog sinking into the cove was the strength that got us back up the hill after 16 hours on the lake. Her 12-quart cast iron cauldron sat on dad's homemade grate, six inches over a bed of split oak, buried in the ground and surrounded by a repurposed steel wheel off a Caterpillar road grader. Like a pot of lava, a fat bubble surfaced every few minutes.

Dick, Gary, Cooder and I arrived on Friday for setup. We took the sunrise patrol on Saturday to ensure all systems were go. By noon, 2-3 boatloads of friends arrived at our campsite on the shores of the 26-mile-long lake.

The Amazing Dick Bass did not come by his moniker casually. He was a skilled musician, a Ph.D. and pioneer in the field of alternative transportation. He served in soup kitchens and homeless shelters and was one of the finest Christians I have ever met. That said, as long as I had known him he had been a bit envious of Kermit the Frog. When your brow creased and before you could ask, he would grin, "because he could squat right down on a lily pad and play his banjo."

One of the most selfless humans I have ever known, this moment was all his.

The Cat Dancer and crew were running on empty and the spicy aroma of campfire and cayenne drifted from the trees near camp. As we returned to Paradise Cove to retrieve Dick and the others, I was wholly unprepared for the scene. The inlet had become a flotilla of quarter-million dollar house boats, Ski Nautiques and jon boats. We idled through the crowd seeking our deserted crew, only to find Professor Bass center stage and solo.

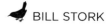 BILL STORK

Propped on a foam float and a black rubber inner tube, he sported white swim trunks with a brown stripe down the side and streaks of Coppertone.

Banjo on his knee and bandage on his head, he deftly fielded requests for bluegrass classics he had known since birth and radio pop songs he had only heard. Sunburned and soaked, folks of all ages were clogging and clapping, dancing and singing on the decks of their floating mobile homes, the sandy shoreline and in their inner tubes. Kids doing Tarzan yells as they dropped off the rope swing provided the crowd noise.

He looked up through his gold rimmed glasses — half-cocked, water-splashed, and taped, smiled with his whole head and drawled:

"Billy Stork, Kermit the Frog ain't got nothin' on me today!" ⋙

The Austin Brisket Debacle of 1994

If ever there is a time when Wisconsin is less than paradise, it would be late February/early March. Having fought through the teeth of winter, still weeks before green grass, I booked a ticket to the Live Music Capitol of the World, Austin, Texas.

My nomadic friend Arlin Rodgers was more than cordial. Willing to take a break from unlocking the mechanisms of liver cancer to play host and music guide, he intended to establish himself as a real Texan by having homemade barbecue upon arrival.

Predictably, the day of departure brought cows with calving difficulty, twisted stomachs and weather the likes of which had never been seen before, or since. Our driveway and every runway in the Midwest was buried by 6" of granular ice.

Failure was not an option. As we found the only plane flying on Thursday February 27, 1994, Dr. Rodgers tended the beef brisket. With cell-phones and email in their infancy and texting not yet imagined, our hero flexed with our unknown arrival, adjusting the heat with precision, one briquette at a time...

The mesquite clung to Arlin's sweatshirt as we wedged into the cab of his Chevy S-10, named Emmitt. Parched and ravenous, we salivated like Pavlov's dogs. Ten minutes seemed an eternity to South Congress Avenue. Deaf to the din pouring from the Continental Club, only a Shiner Bock and a heaping plate of barbecue would fill this void.

As Emmitt growled up the long driveway, we could see mesquite curling from the vent hole in the Weber One-Touch that incubated the King's Cut of Texas Barbecue.

Reunion banter would wait; it was time to feast. With trepidation, Dr. Rodgers presented our smoked centerpiece. The smell was pure hill-country Texas, but that's when the wheels fell off.

The Ginsu knife may be able to effortlessly slice tin cans, but was no match for this roasted cow flank.

 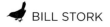 BILL STORK

Admittedly, when we were able to detach a bite-sized piece the flavor was perfect. To chew and swallow, however, was to risk irreparable damage to one's TMJ or an esophageal foreign body. Had I sewn a slab to the sole of my Red Wing work boot, it would surely be there today.

I love Arlin like a brother. He has introduced me to music that has changed my life, and stood by me twice, during the most difficult times. We routinely demonstrate affection by knowing the other's weakness, and skillfully, relentlessly teasing one another.

That being the case, on that day and in the years since, I said nothing — either because some things are simply too sacred or because the most effective form of abuse is to say nothing.

Deliberately, cowardly, I avoided comparison by not attempting my own brisket for 18 years.

Well Arf, you are free. While today I created the second-best, most flavorful, tender and moist brisket in history, I cheated. Sure, the last hour was on the coals, but the first two were in a fully digital pressure cooker. ⬅️

Hedley Can Swim Clear 'Cross

To anyone who has ever considered writing in any form, I implore you to do so, whether it be a diary that that lives in the second drawer of your nightstand or a New York Times best seller. You will at least resurrect thoughts that had escaped for decades, if not learn things about yourself and others that you had never known.

In the two years these ramblings have been published I can think of few, if any times, when that was not the case. I can think of none more so than the one to follow. This is the story of a dog named Hedley, and my friend Dr. Bruce Rummenie.

Bruce was born and raised in Quincy, Illinois, on the shores of the mighty Mississippi, some 480 river miles upstream from Memphis. He studied at the University of Illinois, Urbana-Champaign, reminiscent of the east side of Madison, land-locked by corn fields rather than Lake Monona. Upon graduation, he didn't go far. He took a job in the Urbana School district as an eighth grade English teacher. Minus one year in the late eighties, he has yet to leave.

Never to be mistaken for Austin, Texas, Champaign nonetheless had no shortage of study breaks and live music. Within earshot of the student union and the iconic *Alma Mater* statue, was Mecca. 36 stairs up, overlooking the 600 block of East Green Street was Mabel's, a black cave, capacity 365. In my eight years at the University of Illinois, Mabel's hosted the likes of the Red Hot Chili Peppers, REM, Anson Funderburgh, and The Black Crowes. Near midnight on September 22, 1985, Neil Young, Willy Nelson, Bob Dylan, John Fogerty and Mellencamp, B.B. King, Bon Jovi, and most of the line-up from Farm Aid graced the tiny stage for an after-hours show.

On October 21, 1986 we left Townsend 2South to celebrate our friend Jay Walker's 21st birthday. The lineup at Mabel's that night started with a funk and pop band called the Modern Humans. The night would be headlined by an indie rock outfit called Otis and the Elevators, fronted by a future orthopedic surgeon, with a physical chemist on bass. In the middle was a retro Texas Blues and swing outfit named after the minor league baseball team from the

80 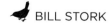 BILL STORK

hometown of Corporal Maxwell Klinger, The Mudhens. Little did I know the music that night would become the soundtrack of our adolescence and beyond. The friends would be brothers, 'til death do us part. The man on lead guitar would become a mentor.

The Mudhens were: Ricky "the fever" Cummings, the world's most polite drummer who transported his equipment on a trailer behind his BMW motorcycle; Scott "the boy wonder" Portzline on bass, the man who would eventually bring you all things with the Nike "swoosh"; Kevin Deforrest, lead singer, a 6ft 7inch Olympic swimmer with a gravel bucket baritone and a gift for gab (think Michael Phelps with shoulder length waves and a Skoal ring meets John Lee Hooker).

Finally, there was Bruce. Monday through Friday, Bruce Rummenie shaped young minds with grammar and composition. On Saturday nights he strapped on a blonde '62 Fender Strat belt buckle high and carpenter level, plugged into a Fender Twin Reverb. He stepped up to a microphone, closed both eyes and let 'er fly. From that moment forward, Bruce Rummenie became, "The Bruiser Man."

Bruiser wrote and sang songs about girls and God. The difference was seldom clear. You would describe Bruiser's faith in the same breath as his height, weight, and age. It was never out front or confrontational, and never did he preach or profess. Rather it was woven into the lyrics of his songs, often by way of double entendre: "All my heart, all my soul, all of my mind, I want to love you," would make a fitting profession of love to a potential mate. The title of the song is *Deuteronomy*.

It was in the way he carried himself. After wreaking havoc on a Saturday night juke joint with nothing more than a six string guitar and twelve bar blues, he met high fives and handshakes with a sheepish glance in the general direction of the floor, "Thanks man, 'preciate that."

It was in the way he listened: slightly slouched, brow deeply creased and his hand covering his mouth. When talking with Bruiser you were moved to speak slowly and think; to fully consider the plight and position of your fellow man of whom you speak.

Born and raised in the back pew of 8:00 Mass and CCD, I didn't realize the man who would help quietly carry my faith from apron strings to adulthood would regularly hold court over a writhing dance floor in a college bar.

When there was celebrating to do, there was only one call to make.

When there was bread and water to be presented to the Altar at a Catholic service, the number was the same.

At a time when I found myself in a place deep, dark, and without a glimmer of hope, I reached out to the Bruiser. His answer was in my mailbox in 24 hours.

With his band The Javelina's, he recorded an album called *All I know*; thirteen songs from a man who had also known pain. Seven songs of commiseration, with titles like "Pain as Big as Texas," and "Home is where the Heartbreaks," followed by 6 songs of hope, with titles like "Love in the Light" and "Let me be your Pony." Where once there was not a glimmer, there was now an Olympic torch at the end of the tunnel.

For all that Bruiser was as a Christian, an educator and a musician, the circle was made complete by a 6-year-old black and white collie. If ever there was a pair who clearly demonstrated the symbiosis between man and beast, it was Bruce and Hedley.

By 1991, Bruiser had woven his presence into the musical and poetic fabric of Champaign-Urbana for the better part of a decade. Yet, he found himself without a band — neither to accompany his guitar and vocals, nor, more importantly, to adorn his left hand. He petitioned the school district for a sabbatical and loaded his blue Toyota 4x4 with three Fenders, a hollow body Gibson, and a Fender Twin Reverb. Hedley rode shotgun.

Two tanks of fuel and a potty break found them in Dallas where they filled up on unleaded and brisket. Past Waco, three and a half hours later, they rolled onto 6th Street, Austin Texas. Bruiser had twelve months to shop his chops around the live music capitol of the world, and maybe find a date.

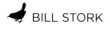 BILL STORK

It's been said the guitar player always gets the girl; so far that hadn't held up, due in no small part to his nature. Though he had written songs to the contrary, Bruiser was in search of Mrs. Right, and had little interest in Miss Right Now. As history will account, his wingman Hedley was bound by no such principles.

Austin is the incubator of all things liberal in the Great Republic of Texas. The live music scene is traced to a gas station owned by Kenneth Threadgill, opening in 1933. *Threadgills* has grown into an iconic restaurant and music venue that routinely hosts the likes of Kris Kristofferson and Willie Nelson around a big oak table, over their famous chicken fried steak. In 1960, Threadgill himself pushed a young singer in front of the microphone, and so began the ultimately tragic career of Janis Joplin.

The de facto Mayor of Austin is a Chicago-born, Jewish country singer named Kinky Friedman who pulled 12% of the votes in the 2006 gubernatorial election. The town motto, official or not is, "keep Austin weird," and bar time is according to one Clifford Antone (1949-2006), the proprietor of the club that gave birth to the likes of the Fabulous Thunderbirds and Stevie Ray Vaughn.

There is more music in Austin at 5:00 on a Tuesday afternoon than Chicago on a Saturday night, and leash laws are of little concern. So, a guitar man with a case full of Freddy King, and a collie with an independent streak longer than his nose were set.

Nearing the end of four years of veterinary school, spring break found me a little tired in the head and missing my friend Bruiser. With gas just over a buck a gallon and my Bronco II getting nearly 25 miles per, I figured a hundred dollars would get us there and back. A thousand miles didn't seem so far for a little barbecue, a whole lot of music, and a Shiner Bock.

If we drove to St. Louis on a Wednesday, we could get a free meal and a bed at my friend Jeff Slaby's, and easily make Austin for the first note, Thursday night at Joe's Generic Bar. My friend, native Texan, and protagonist of "The Great Austin Brisket Debacle" Arlin Rogers, my 6-month-old lab Cooder, and I loaded 150 CDs and two bags of nacho cheese Corn Nuts, and we were gone.

His first roadtrip since being adopted from the animal shelter, Cooder was amazing. His bladder held as long as ours but when we fell into Bruiser's driveway and Cooder's feet hit the ground, he was ready to rip. With nearly 24 hours' worth of puppy to burn, he commenced hot laps around the cottage, butt tucked low for stability, back legs reaching past his nose. With Arlin as my witness, the gravel hadn't settled from the second lap when he was coming around for the third.

On lap four, he noticed Hedley on the front porch. Next time around, he dropped his landing gear and came to a dusty, skidding stop, studying the collie. Hedley kept his head between his paws, body slightly curved, never so much as lifting his head. It would appear that haggard travelers and maniacal yellow puppies are routine in Hedley's world.

Cooder turned to get our take on the situation; Arlin and I shrugged. Cooder trotted onto the porch, and took his place next to Hedley. When in Rome, you do as the Romans; when in Austin, you chill.

Midway through his time in Austin, Bruiser found himself in a familiar place, a thousand miles south of home. It has been said "the blues is all about feelin' good, about feelin' bad." With his Jimmy Vaughn and T-Bone Walker licks Bruiser had no trouble finding a stage, and the people loved him. But affairs of the heart, still elusive.

Austin's climate lends itself to screen doors, with humidity that tends to warp them so that they no longer latch. That worked nicely for Hedley. More socially comfortable than Bruiser, when the weather was nice Hedley would let himself out to go visiting.

Once, while out for a stroll with Bruiser along the Colorado River, Hedley was rushed by a young family. Obviously familiar, Hedley dropped to a play-bow and chased the young boys around the statue of Stevie Ray Vaughn. Looking a bit awkward, the parents extended a hand to Bruiser, "oh, you must be Hedley's dad."

Around that time Hedley had fallen into a pattern of excusing himself nearly every evening, not to return until the middle of the next morning. Bruiser could not help but be concerned, if not curious.

 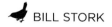 BILL STORK

One morning, Bruiser was out on a run. A few blocks from home, a screen door creaked. Onto the porch strode the vision of a University of Texas student's dream. One step behind was Hedley. He slowed just enough so she could lean down to plant a soft kiss on his long nose.

Down the steps, he fell in next to Bruiser. Side by side, stride for stride, they completed the 3-mile loop.

It was abundantly clear. The title of "Master" had passed from man to beast. ❧

Hedley Rides Again

You may recall my friend Bruiser, the God-fearing guitar slinger from Champaign, Illinois, his venerable collie Hedley and their adventures during a sabbatical in Austin.

For those of us old enough to recall 8-track tapes and dial phones, we may also remember the early incarnations of the Toyota pickup truck. Famous for two things: you could change the oil the day your son was baptized, then not again until he was an ordained Catholic priest; and the engine would tick along silent as a Singer sewing machine. All the while, the wheel wells would start to rust before the plastic was off the seats the day you brought it home from the dealer.

Bruiser had a blue "extended cab." Long before "Mega" and "King," there may have been enough room behind the driver's seat for a set of jumper cables and a sandwich, so long as it wasn't a Dagwood Bumstead model. For ventilation it had a sliding rear window, the latch having broken years previous.

As groupies who didn't know a bar chord from a blues riff, we would help carry the equipment down the stairs and load the truck. Bruiser was equal parts utilitarian and methodical. We soon learned for the PA speakers and the bass amp to set the edges against the cab and tailgate, and the mic stands, chords, boards and instruments filled in the middle.

The Toyota 4x4 would haul either the lead guitar player, singer and all the equipment for a 5-piece Texas Blues band, or Hedley.

If not mentioned previously, Hedley had horrible thunderstorm phobia. His coping mechanisms primarily involved going around — or through — whatever separated him from the freshly planted arugula in Bruiser's garden, and digging it up.

One afternoon in June, what had separated him from the garden was the screen in the storm door. A few weeks later Bruiser had collected a long enough list to justify a trip to Ace Hardware, so he loaded the broken door and Hedley into the back of the Toyota. Partly cloudy and cool, it was a perfect day for a drive.

 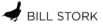 BILL STORK

I've only received mail in two states, and they're only separated by a toll booth and allegiance to conference rivals in the NFL. Yet, every place I've been, some barista, bartender or bike mechanic will cackle like it's the first time anyone's ever said, "If you don't like the weather, just wait 10 minutes, it'll change." I'll get to England someday. I've heard the only thing worse than the weather is the food, and neither has changed for centuries. Possibly this explains why American blues are so well received in London.

In the ten minutes from home to hardware, partly cloudy and cool became a respectable downpour. Rather than wait for his driver to come to his senses, Hed used his collie nose like a flat blade screwdriver, wedged open the sliding window and dove into the comfort of the cab where by his (and our) way of thinking, he belonged anyway. Moving his wipers from intermittent to low, Bruiser couldn't get overly upset at the dripping dog in his passenger seat.

The rain was reasonable and Bruiser young and fleet, so he respectfully passed the open spot near the front door, and took a head-in spot twenty yards from the entrance. Minutes later he had lugged the screen door — with a hole the exact dimensions of a collie, like Wile E. Coyote's outline — into the store.

Before the helpful hardware man could assess, however, an announcement came through the intercom:

"Would the owner of the blue Toyota please come to the front of the store, immediately." He was not comforted by the small crowd pressed against the store window, pointing and aghast.

Faster than the automatic sliding door, he nearly head-planted the glass, as, knees shaking he burst onto the sidewalk to see what had happened. The rain had ramped to monsoon intensity. Hedley had switched from passenger to driver's seat, and in doing so, he bumped the gearshift. In neutral and weighing little more than a Jersey cow, the truck rolled passed the car parked next to it. Without so much as touching a yellow line, in a gentle arc the truck slid perfectly into the open space near the front door.

Oblivious to his audience, Hedley sat behind the wheel, surveying his new view.

On a bench outside the Jo Ann Fabric next door, an elderly gentleman sat, hands folded over the head of his cane. Waiting for Bruiser to catch his senses, he cackled, "Between you and me young man, your dog drives a heck of a lot better than my wife."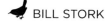

Dr. Ryan

Life in general, and veterinary school in particular, will bring you into acquaintance with amazing people. I'm working on a theory that if you dig a little, most people are. Being most familiar with the University of Illinois class of 1992, we'll start there.

In the University of Illinois class of 1992, we had Joe Whalen, who is a far superior veterinarian and college quarterback than limousine driver, along with "Natural" Dave Rosen, the second ranked light heavy weight kickboxer in the world, and "Sparks" Revenaugh, a Seattle street musician who is now a premier equine specialist. Not to be forgotten are a former Marine, a Cajun Chef, a half dozen farmers, a beer truck driver from Chicago... and Chris Ryan.

Not dissimilar to any rite of passage or apprenticeship, in four years of Veterinary school your world gets pretty small. You become familiar with every water fountain, vending machine and pair of chairs that can be pushed together for a seven minute nap, memorizing the cracks in the concrete path between basic sciences and the clinic.

One day Chris asked if I knew of any good ponds nearby. After six years in Champaign-Urbana and having worked in a tackle store only 40 minutes away, I was primed to help my friend.

"Dr. Nelson has a great little pond with a lot of nice bass, and there is one by Mahommet with some slab-sized crappie, guaranteed." I held out my hand using my fingers to mark Interstates 72 and 74, making Sharpie dots on my palm to mark the exact locations of the little lakes so he could drive straight there.

"If you have a little more time there is a pond over by Farmer City that has some beautiful blue gills," I finished.

Always polite, he drawled, "Ahh Bill, I really appreciate it, but that's a lot of work. Which one is best for sittin' next to, drinkin' a beer, and takin' a nap?"

It may have taken a half-pot of espresso roast and a Red Bull to rev Chris all the way up to laid back, but he was a man of clear purpose and three priorities: veterinary medicine, anything involving a ball, and sleep.

A diligent student, 20 years later he is an outstanding agent of animal health and welfare in "the hog capital of the world."

As for sports, you could invent a new one over breakfast and Chris would kick your butt after lunch. Like Happy Gilmore in surgical scrubs, he would take one full step sideways, and drive a golf ball into next semester. Lob him a softball and he would crank it into the nearest cow pasture simply so he didn't have to run so fast around the bases. Which is not to say he couldn't.

Then, there was sleep. Power naps, catnaps, or seven-minute naps were for rookies. Dr. Ryan scheduled his sleep with the commitment and conviction of national board exams or kidney dialysis:

"Hey Chris, the Dallas Cowboys Cheerleaders are going to be serving free Guinness and bacon cheeseburgers at Murphy's on May 5th!"

May 5th may have been three weeks in the future, but it was after a long stretch of final exams.

"Ahh Bill, I really appreciate the offer, but I'm gonna be sleeping then."

On May 15, 1992 we crossed the stage at the Krannert Center for the Performing Arts, shook hands with former Marine Dr. Erwin Small, who was anything but, and accepted our diplomas. We raised our right hands in oath, switched our tassels from left to right, and where students had stood were 78 newly graduated veterinarians. Some moved to Wisconsin, some back to school to specialize.

Chris went to Henry County, Illinois, a bucolic heartland potpourri of agriculture both new and old, and home to a number of Amish farms. By way of dedication, demeanor and skill-set, Chris was exquisitely suited to serve the community, or so it would seem.

By my way of thinking, one of the best ways to insure maximum productivity is to have some sort of a victory lap at the end of the day; a small ritual that separates the hard thinking, labor, and

 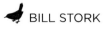 BILL STORK

responsibilities, and dinner with the kids. There is an art and science to it. Bike rides, runs and Pilates are a bonus, but energetically expensive and time consumptive. Not dissimilar to the aforementioned seven minute nap, the little release needs to be significant enough to feel rewarded, but doable on a daily basis. For those who serve in an on-call emergency capacity, there needs to be a "safety" built in.

One Monday evening, Dr. Ryan strolled to his mailbox, pinky wrapped around a Budweiser longneck in the hand that cradled the day's mail, faded flannel shirt untucked, unbuttoned and flapping in the breeze. As he flipped through solicitations from the alumni association and flyers from Kohl's, he stopped dead in his black leather work boots.

A plain white postcard, with letters bolded and blocked, "DOC, COME QUICK, COW HAVING TROUBLE CALVING." Yoder farm.

Even for an unflappable man of medicine, there will be conundrums. Through rain, snow, sleet and hail, the United States Postal Service will deliver. However, they will not move an envelope six inches on Sunday, under any circumstances. It had been at least two days since the snail mail smoke signal had been sent. He scrolled through his experience and education trying to imagine what could still be as urgent Monday evening as on Saturday before noon.

He was scheduled to be in the area the next morning, so he planned to leave early. To his understanding, the Amish were not prone to ambush; still he was a bit apprehensive as he approached the iconic red hip-roof barn, just as the sun rose. It did nothing for his wonder as a horde of formally dressed children swarmed his truck as he rolled into the door yard. Nearly pulling the door off his Ford Courier the kids bantered, "oh thank you, thank you for coming so quickly."

The children's gratitude was trumped only by the look of helplessness in the big brown eyes of the crossbred Jersey. From her back side protruded a calf, bawling and sucking, oblivious to the novelty of her first three days of life. Birtha was quite ready to be done with it.

The cow had begun to deliver on Saturday morning, but when she progressed to pushing the calf's pelvis through her own, they became locked like a 3-D puzzle. Never satisfied with the obvious, veterinary taxonomists call this "hip locked."

For 72 hours without rest, the children had diligently propped three bales of straw under the calf each time the cow stood, and removed them when she lay back down.

Dr. Ryan scuffed his Tingley rubber overshoes on the barn lime and paused. He stroked his whiskers and nodded as if that's the way it happens every day. He walked to his little truck and returned with an epidural, lube and a calf-puller

Minutes later, he had delivered the last quarter of the calf. The children rejoiced, Birtha was relieved, and the vet is still shaking his head, 20 years later. 🐦

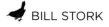 BILL STORK

When Love Comes to Town

Inspired by the global success of Live Aid, conceived to bring awareness to the ongoing famine in Ethiopia, Willie Nelson, John Mellencamp and Neil Young organized a movement to bring aid and awareness to the struggling American Family Farmer.

Farm Aid I took place on September 22, 1985, in Champaign, Illinois. The iconic lineup ranged from Texas songwriter Joe Elly to the Mount Rushmore of Country Music: Waylon Jennings, Willie Nelson, Johnny Cash and Kris Kristofferson. Performing at 10:00 a.m. may have been wholly out of character for Bon Jovi and Tom Petty, but they held nothing back. Few will forget Billy Joel's maniacal 22 minutes, on piano, vocals and at least 3 pots of coffee.

There were 44 acts, each one a giant in their genre, and that day they brought it all. Ask any of the 80,000 of us who were there soaked and frozen for 14 hours and every note to name the single most enduring moment, and half, without hesitation, will say BB King.

Six days past his 60th birthday, navy blue 3-piece suit and tie, center stage. With Lucille strapped high around his neck and a football stadium in the palm of his hand, he eased into, "The Thrill is Gone." Let the record show that day, and two and a half decades to follow, nothing could be further from the truth.

With a Hammond B-3 organ underpinning the urgency, he pined "I'll still live on baby... but how lonely I'll be." With 80,000 people feelin' the pain, he dropped his head, pulled his elbows tight and Lucille close. He launched one of his trademark guitar sermons. As he paused to bend his bottom three strings and tug at your soul, his B-string snapped.

Oblivious to the driving rain, without pause or opening his eyes, he slipped out a replacement string. With a few whole notes and three soft choruses of "the thrill is gone" from the congregation swaying in synchrony, clapping the down-beats, the '58 Gibson was restrung, tuned. Before the thunderous applause would quiet, the undisputed King of the Blues and master showman launched.

As if to demonstrate that "the blues is all about feeling good, about feeling bad," he romped through "Let the Good Times Roll" and took every last one of us with him.

Ten years later I was blessed to be able to ring in 1996 with a dozen of my best friends, and BB King. By then he sat through most of his shows but what he lost as a performer was gained as a statesman. He was the headliner, and in charge to be certain. The venue was the magnificent Grand Central Station in Chicago, but we had arrived early and were close enough that we could touch his wingtips. My vision of midnight was a beaming BB, sitting and strumming rhythm as two of his disciples, Sonny Landreth and John Hiatt worked the crowd and their instruments.

It is without an ounce of overstatement that BB King has deeply influenced everyone who has strapped on and plugged in an electric guitar since 1950. Through the middle of his career, he averaged over 250 appearances per year, and in 1956 played an exhausting 342 shows. He has performed for presidents, won 15 Grammies in 4 categories, medals of freedom and art heritage, been awarded honorary doctorates, and decorated from Portland, Maine, to Stockholm, Sweden. He was unanimously voted into the Blues and Rock and Roll Halls of Fame.

Not to be overlooked is that his career spanned decades when James Hood was denied entrance to the University of Alabama, and Rosa Parks was expected to sit in the back of a bus. As our country struggled to integrate, artists like BB, Willie Nelson, Ray Charles and the great Earl Scruggs were famously and demonstrably color blind. He appeared and recorded with countless artists ranging from the Rolling Stones to Eric Clapton and U2.

After a show on the campus of the University of Illinois, a good friend wanted to meet the man, hoping his son would absorb the history he had just witnessed, while still in utero. His wife Kim was eight months pregnant, and feeling anything but attractive. For her, the thrill was indeed gone. Familiar with the auditorium, we knocked on the stage door, which promptly opened. A handler nodded with a smile and promised that he would ask.

BILL STORK

In minutes the door opened again, and there stood "The King of the Blues." Kevin was composed, if not original. He shook hands and clasped the elbow of BB King, unfazed that he had sweat through his sport coat in the course of the 90-minute show. Kevin thanked him for all that his music had meant to him, and how cool it was when he changed a string in the middle of a solo during Farm Aid.

As if he had no place to be, Mr. King smiled graciously and asked where we were from, and what we did for a living. As we answered, Kim tried to make herself small; not easy for a woman within weeks of delivering a baby, as she drifted a half step back at the end of the line.

Politely and without breaking conversation, BB wiped his hands on a white cloth flung over his shoulder, and dropped to one knee before Kim. He covered her left hand with both his hands, looked up at the expectant and particularly self-conscious mother and spoke softly, "little lady, they ain't nothin' in the world more beautiful than a pregnant woman."

BB King has been recognized and voted among the best and most influential artists and guitarists of our time. Which only serves to magnify his grace and humility. BB is a credit to his race... the human race. ◆

Olé

It was early spring 1985, at South Farms, University of Illinois. Late in the third year of my undergraduate education, I pondered my future. Having recently attended a local rodeo and seen the *Running of the Bulls* in Pamplona on TV, rodeo clown and matador were looking pretty good. Thanks to a deep thigh bruise and a gash in my pride, the dogged pursuit of a DVM would be right back on track.

The University of Wisconsin has the Memorial Union Terrace where students can relax with a fine beverage and watch the sunset over Lake Mendota, while listening to live reggae and blues bands. The basketball and hockey Badgers compete in the Kohl Center, and the football team in iconic Camp Randall Stadium.

While claiming no superiority, at the University of Illinois we had the South Farms. A soft spring breeze through a biology lecture would remind students that just beyond the Assembly Hall were two farrow-to-finish swine operations, a sheep farm, a cow calf operation and a horse farm.

In Chemistry 101 you titrate acids and bases wearing safety glasses and a white coat. In Agriculture classes, you're gonna get organic, to the extent that your political science roommate may meet you at the door with a towel and a bar of soap. That said, they never failed to be eventful.

Four hours before 80,000 people would descend upon Memorial Stadium for the first Farm Aid concert, I was returning from lamb watch for my small ruminant class. Well before 9-11 security, I rode my bike through the gates and past the stage. In the pre-dawn fog a man, guitar on his knee, was singing "Knocking on Heaven's Door."

Thirty years later, a personal concert by Bob Dylan is a story to tell. At 21, doing calf check with Becky Bull was way more current.

You can say there are Ag majors, and there are farm kids. The former, I grew up in a town of 100,000 and worked at the Brush College Animal Hospital cleaning cages and surgical instruments.

 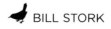 BILL STORK

I counted minnows and night crawlers at Dave's Tackle Box and spent ten days on my uncle's beef farm. The latter, Becky grew up on an Angus farm, and showed cattle at the North American International Livestock Exposition.

By grace and good fortune, Becky and I were paired to check the cow herd as a unit of Beef Production 101. It was mid-April, 45F, and driving rain. She showed up in a cherry red F-350, with snow plow bracket, search lights and a grille the size of a movie screen. In the back was a 50-gallon diesel tank and galvanized tool box the width of the bed. She could do a C-section, brand a herd of cattle, or overhaul a John Deere 4020 without going to town.

I drove my grandma's 1974 Plymouth Valiant, and brought a flashlight.

As we walked the pasture, occasionally a cow and calf would saunter through the high beams trained on as much of the landscape as we could capture. Bolts of lightning would flash the herd for unpredictable seconds at a time. Our flashlights were futile, as driving rain reflected the light right back at our retinas. As close as we could tell, everyone outside was ok. By our way of thinking, if there was action, it would be in the corn stalk bedding in the back of the lean-tos.

Half an hour in a rainstorm had only served to feature the Macon County *Fairest of the Fair*, 1983, at her finest. Seed cap backwards, hair tucked behind her ears, her thousand-watt smile and aqua green eyes shone like a café sign to a road-weary trucker.

As we passed under the shelter, the breath of a dozen cows, and thoughts of Becky, fogged my glasses instantly. Not more than three steps in, on my left flank appeared a white head, and I was launched like a beach ball at a Buffet concert by a 1200-pound Hereford who was minutes post-partum.

Seconds before liftoff, my mind had been racing as to how I might segue calf watch into coffee and a donut. For the duration of flight, I was equally preoccupied, hoping my fingers would find space between the corrugated tin and the 2x6 cross member that supported the structure, lest I was assured another volley or two.

As I clung to the wall and a sliver of dignity, the cow pawed the bedding and snorted, as if I didn't get the message.

For Becky, it was just another day at the office. She squared her shoulders and raised her arms like a flagman at the finish of the Daytona 500. Summoning her inner Aretha Franklin, she pulled up a deep growl, "C'mon Na, You girls GIT! on outa heeaah and let that po' boy down off the wall."

Like a kid caught in the cookie jar, Hereford cow, ear tag 487, dropped her head in apology and ambled back to her baby. Trembling, I let myself back to the ground.

"You ok?" Becky deadpanned.

Copping her calm, I brushed myself off and shrugged, loosely alluding to my lack of vision, and answered "Oh yeah, no problem."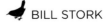

BILL STORK

Abby to the Rescue

Some names in this story have been changed to protect anonymity. Artistic license may have been taken in order to make characters seem as great as they truly are.

Three hundred sixty four days a year, well before dawn cracks through the cul-de-sac, Abby the Westie is all about business and breakfast. Through her back yard and just past the lilacs, there is an 80-year-old retired teacher eternally grateful that on one eventful day, she deviated.

Thanks to Terrier Tenacity, a chemical engineer who can't handle his Kool-Aid, and an orthopedic surgeon skilled with scalpel and Fender Stratocaster yet agile enough to dodge a 9-iron, Irene Renfro is today trading her walker for a crutch.

First, a little background…

Danny Cane arrived at the University of Illinois in 1981. He had earned enough Advanced Placement credit in high school to technically qualify as a professor. When I came to know him two years later, he had forever assumed the moniker of his home town of Red Bud, Illinois, and his forehead was beginning to overtake his red hairline.

At 5'9" and 180 lbs he could best be described as a carrot-topped, chemical engineering equivalent of the Tasmanian Devil, with only slightly better table manners. Having lived only a few doors down in Townsend Residence Hall, I can speak from experience. The man walked fast, ate fast, read books fast, showered quickly, and I am convinced he even slept fast. Long ago I developed the highly functional habit of memorizing the cars people drive and the shoes they wear. It provides a little insight as to their personality and function and helps me remember names. You can tell from the road if a friend is at the hardware store or pub and you can speak topically to the person on the other side of the bathroom stall divider. Red Bud Cane wasted no time on the groover.

The morning of Sunday, October 10, 1986, however, he moved slowly. Very slowly.

October 9, 1986 was the 21st birthday of my friend whose parents named him after a pedestrian traffic violation. It was a Saturday night and The Mudhens were opening for Otis and the Elevators. It was time to mobilize the ranks and celebrate with Jay Walker.

On stage, The Elevators was a jam band, long before Dave Mathews and Phish, and devoid of anyone named Otis. They were well known for their perpetual hypnotic danceable grooves, and the guitar work of one Jim Bury. A card-carrying disciple of Stevie Ray Vaughn, Jim could let it fly. He lined spare picks on his microphone stand and wore a feather on the head of his guitar. Minus the floor-length robe, even his stance was SRV.

Mabel's Bar was tended by a good friend and future colleague named "Natural" Dave Rosen. Grateful for my having saved him from a life as a lawyer, he refused to charge me or anyone I had ever known for a beer. Through four years of veterinary school, Dave was the third-ranked full contact karate fighter in the world. With hands soft to nurture a newborn kitten yet hard and swift to render a competitor comatose, he could spin a long neck Budweiser on each knuckle, bump them on the bar and spin the caps into the garbage or the upper deck.

On this momentous night, Red Bud decided to join us. Though a St. Louis Cardinal fan from birth, and having grown up just across the Mississippi from the Budweiser Brewery, he didn't much care for beer. Not to fear, I explained to Dave that Red Bud was a cautious consumer and he brewed up a tasty purple punch, right before our eyes.

The ultimate moment in most Otis shows was usually in the second encore, and long after bar time. Jim would pull his pearl top Strat close to his body, tuck his elbows in, rock back on his heels, drop his head, and kick it off. With Mark "Toupee" Zehr on bass they would lay down the groove and, in one writhing mass, the crowd would move. After ten minutes of soaring guitar and in a fashion Mother Goose could have never intended, he would hammer a chord, the band would pause, crowd go silent and Jim would attack the microphone, "Mary had a little lamb, his fleece was black as coal, yeah..." And the crowd went wild.

 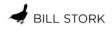 BILL STORK

Jim once told me, "Bill, if you stand on your head every night, you got nothin' left for the next show." Like his mentor, Jim would always leave us begging for just a little bit more.

Having properly celebrated Jay, but being the academics we were, mid-terms loomed. So we filtered to the street below. Thankfully, it was an easy quarter mile down Green Street, past the statue of the Alma Mater back to the dorm. Our teetotaling chemical genius Red Bud needed a little guidance, a couple of shoulders and a few breaks. Dave's purple punch had hit him hard.

In hindsight, I did feel a twinge of guilt. At breakfast the next morning we watched him try and hold his head in a way that didn't hurt, all the while swearing never to do it again, and hoping the bacon grease, scrambled eggs and shredded cheese would displace or absorb the toxins inflaming his brain.

My intention was always to tell him that Dave's concoction was Welch's Grape Juice and a splash of 7-Up, on the rocks.

As for Otis and the Elevators, they would gig from Champaign, Illinois, to the University of Wisconsin Memorial Union Terrace. Well before the Internet and satellite radio, they had to do things the hard way. By invitation, Jim Bury would strap on Bono's guitar and jam with The Edge when U2 came to town. They opened for, and Jim hosted, a clean and sober Stevie Ray.

Their breakout involved a dilapidated appliance truck with their old gear and a west coast tour from Seattle to LA. Otis and the Elevators recorded two acclaimed records (yes, 33.3 rpm vinyl records). They came close, but never "made" it.

If there was to be a future and families, it was time to turn to book learning. On a spectacular spring day, Jim was golfing with his mother. The ninth green overlooked Lake of the Woods and the fairways were Ireland green. As she lined up an easy 10-foot putt, he puffed his chest and spoke the words any parent would live to hear:

"Mom, I've decided to quit the band, and go to medical school."

In a made-for-Caddyshack moment, she froze like a Macy's mannequin, and asked him to repeat.

His head cocked slightly, he inflected a statement with a question mark: "Mom, I've been accepted into medical school...?"

She inhaled, coiled and came out swinging. He ducked like a Golden Gloves boxer. The young bluesman was fleet, but mom was fuming like Yosemite Sam. Once he was out of her strike zone, she let the putter fly and did not stop until she had emptied every club from her bag. Out of clubs, she unzipped the pocket, flung every last golf ball at him, and then kicked her bag.

Hands on her hips, she fumed, "You had a perfectly good career going with the rock and roll band and you want to (excuse me) PISS it all away and be a damn DOCTOR?"

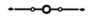

By obligation, and for the better of us all, time marches on. In the quarter century since, Jim Bury, Daniel "Red Bud" Cane and tens of others were not to be heard from, until September 2013.

Retired teacher Irene Renfro is not to be caught in bed when the sun comes up, regardless of the calendar and when dawn gets scheduled. Widowed for decades and retired from a life of education for years, her body is to stay in motion and she will take no chances with an idle mind.

While backing down her driveway, she caught a glimpse of the St. Louis Post Dispatch in her rearview. Rather than run it down, she tapped the brakes and rolled out of her car. Just short of 80, and operating on a couple artificial joints, spry this lady was not.

The driveway sloped just gently enough to flow water to the storm sewer and she had missed "P" on the shifter. As she bent to pick up the paper, the open door hit her in the hinder and funneled her under the car.

Like a scene from a horror movie, the front tire rolled up her pubic bone, rocked back down, and her pelvis became a parking block.

She screamed for help. Unfortunately, even a retired teacher can't generate a lot of decibels with a Nissan Versa resting on her chest. Fortunately, the time of day that Irene is prone to collecting her

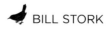 BILL STORK

paper is when Abby the Westie insists on her morning constitutional. (Remember Abby?)

On this day, Abby did not immediately return for her half cup of Fromm's. Rather than risk waking his neighbors, before calling her name, Wolfgram grabbed the Maglite and launched down the back stairs.

He heard his Westie, polite by breed standards, barking like Timmy had fallen in the well.

Moving to the sound, he rounded the lilacs and found his elderly neighbor trapped under her car. He pushed like a lineman on a blocking sled, relieving the pressure on her pelvis. Abby's barks had managed to alert the neighbor, an ER nurse returning from shift, who supported Irene until the EMTs arrived minutes later.

The doctors and nurses at Alton Memorial provided excellent and immediate care. She was stable for the moment, on pain meds and fluids, but a two-ton economy car resting on an octogenarian is a concern. A collapsed lung and lacerated liver got Irene wheeled onto a med flight helicopter.

A stone's-throw over "Big Muddy" and just past Busch Memorial Stadium is Barnes-Jewish Medical Center, known regionally for exceptional patient care and renowned for some of the finest doctors in the world. After repeated imaging, Irene was found to have a fractured pelvis.

Though surgery was an option, Dr. Jim Bury judged that her recovery would be far quicker with excellent pain management, rest and support.

Irene's pain was managed by one of the area's finest, Dr. Daniel ("Red Bud") Cane. ᴥ

Hey, Porter

Comedian and native Ukrainian, Yakov Smirnoff made a career out of glorifying life in America, compared to Russia: "In America you go looking for party; in my country, party looks for you!"

Whether UW or U of I, you did not have to look hard. After a week of quizzes, tests and lab reports, come Friday, brain dead co-eds were ready to shut off.

It could have been my red neck, blue collar or empty wallet, but I couldn't bring myself to go straight from chem lab to quarter beers. My idea of happy hour was to turn the radio up louder than the industrial sterilizer at Noyes Lab. Decades earlier, scientists brought polyester to seventies politicians and John Travolta in the very same building. In 1984, seven hours a week washing rat cages brought a flat-top freshman a little foldin' money and a pepperoni pizza on Sunday night.

I wouldn't make two steps inside the door of Townsend 2-South before my roommate, "Senator" Scott Clewis, would politely hand me a fresh towel and a bar of soap. There must have been something about the smell. By the time I had scrubbed off the animal odor, a crowd would gather in front of the 14" black and white TV in our 20x20 dorm room.

After Waylon Jennings broke into "Waymore's Blues" at the end of another epic episode of "The Dukes of Hazzard." we would march en masse to the cafeteria for supper, fully intent on breaking bread and getting a head start on Monday's bio final. In spite of our most sincere intentions to dive back into academia, word would spread of a band or a house party.

The plan would become: study for a solid hour, <u>then</u> we would go "for just one set," certain we would study more efficiently with a break.

For every good Saturday morning intention, there was a Friday night temptation. If vet school were to be a reality, there had to be lot more studying with purpose, than sleeping it off.

 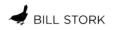 BILL STORK

Intentionally or serendipitously, there was a single factor for me that prevented the perpetual "one more." Through the middle years of my time at University, I had a standing date. At 6:30 sharp every Saturday morning, I met The Amazing Dick Bass at Ye Olde Donut Shop. Thirty years before texting, you made commitments. Bailing or showing up late was never a thought.

Ye Olde Donut Shop was located at the corner of Lincoln Avenue and reality. It was six blocks, two generations and a paradigm away from campus. Figuratively and literally, just south of the railroad tracks. I always realized that our weekly sessions at the donut shop kept me on task, but it wasn't until I had graduated that I came to realize the beauty of the dingy little blue collar pastry shop.

As you walked in, the "fancy" rolls were in a glass case under the counter. On the far wall were rows of the production pastries. There were 8 swivel stools on the long side of the counter, low to the ground so your coattails would brush the floor. It wrapped in the shape of an "L." where there were four more faded maroon and chrome swivels, en route to the facilities.

I always had a chocolate long john and a white iced cake donut and two cartons of milk. ADB was adventurous. He'd have an old fashioned sour cream, and a wild card, usually based on what someone else was having. The coffee cups were full-fledged diner model, white porcelain, inch-thick walls, tapered in the middle.

Two years into our tenure at YODS we had a revelation. I took a bite and stared at the half donut in my hand, "You know, Dick Bass, this place doesn't really have the best donuts in the world."

"Naw, Billy Stork, I reckon I cain't argue with you there.»

"This coffee tastes like ground-up goat hoof."

In front of a classroom or in the laboratory, Dick Bass spoke like the PhD electrical engineer he was. At the donut shop, it was his native Blackshear, Georgia, "Yeah, but you cain't beat the folks."

Katie's smile was worth double the dollar tip a poor college student could leave. It was not as if she wanted to watch the sun rise down Springfield Avenue on Saturday mornings, but she always acted glad to see us.

Dick and I always sat in the middle of the counter, facing "amen" corner. On the wall was Don, the long retired plumber who, by force of habit, sat on the wall opposite the water shed.

The corner stool was reserved for The Rev. "The Reverend" was retired; from what I have no clue. Without fail he would pick a topic from Champaign News Gazette or a snippet of conversation, and he would launch. The "carry out crowd" would smile, and shuffle out the door. Those of us on the long counter would nod.

And so it went, until the day things got personal. The sermon of the day became a full-fledged debate: the Rev claimed The Andy Griffith Show was insulting to rural folk.

I looked to the man on my right. Dick Bass was about to defend his PhD thesis in front of a gallery of General Electric executives. He would become a professor emeritus at Georgia Tech University and revolutionize alternative energy and transportation. He also happened to grow up halfway between Mayberry and Mt. Pilot. The Amazing Dick Bass just smiled.

The fifteen minute dust-up concluded as we laid dollar bills and quarters on the counter for Katie. We shook hands, back slapped and shuffled out smiling.

On any given Saturday you could see folks at the counter looking occasionally over their right shoulder. "Amen corner" looked west down Springfield Avenue. Like it was winking at you with the right headlight, and visible from 6 blocks, the yellow 1977 Lincoln Continental Mark V would roll slowly into the lot.

The door big as a billboard creaked open, and a pair of Allen Edmonds wing tips, spit-shined and polished, would address the pavement. His pace spoke of a man relieved of obligations; his posture of one who had earned it. By the time one of us would open the door, a hush would consume the room.

In retrospect, I wonder what my folks must have thought. Four years at university and thousands in tuition, and the first thing I had to tell them in our Sunday night phone call was a story of an old gentleman at a donut shop. I made it as far as the shoes when Dad interrupted.

 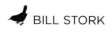 BILL STORK

"Son," he paused to clear some space, "that is Porter Kaise." From 45 miles away through the coiled cord of the old-fashioned land line, you could feel the clench in his fist and the crease in his temples.

"I've worked construction for 30 years and I flat guarantee you that is the finest and fairest human I have ever had the pleasure of working for."

Road construction to romance, "Porter's Pearls" were words to live by.

On affairs of the heart: You need a front po-ach, and a pitcher of ice tea, young man. If you want to get with the girl you jest wait 'til she walks by and say, hey little lady, why don't you come on up here and sit fo'-a-while?

I would borrow a Sharpie from Katie and pull a napkin from the dispenser. The 1985 Ford Bronco II I drove did not exactly ride like a Cadillac Coup de Ville. Anything rougher than a ballroom dance floor, she would rock and roll like a rollercoaster at a small town fair. Having made a mental note, I would ask Porter "Green Street"? He would nod subtly and smile. "Between Randolph and 4th." he specified. I lifted my hand off the words on the napkin, exactly the same.

As my 8800 lb pickup truck heads due East on Hwy 18, the frost heaves rattle her 'til the headlights are headed towards Johnson Creek. It's been 30 years, yet I am still inspired.

I ate fewer than a half dozen donuts and shared a pot of lukewarm pond water with Porter Kaise. A man known as a master of his craft, mentioned in the second breath, after the respect he showed to, and earned from those he worked with. ◅▻

In Practice

BILL STORK

Pumpkin

Twenty-one years ago, I graduated from the University of Illinois – College of Veterinary Medicine. In the process of considering jobs at clinics in most Big Ten states I met a lot of nice people and saw plenty of beautiful, productive land. None could match the lush, green, rolling hills, lakes, rivers and hip-roof dairy barns of southern Wisconsin, so I migrated across the Cheddar Curtain.

This decision I have never regretted; as the years have unfolded it has proven home to the finest folks I am proud to call friends. Call it fate, faith or dumb luck, and it may have taken 17 years to find her, but it is also where the love of my life was born and raised.

In 1992, LMVC kept a satellite clinic on Main Street in Cambridge. One could say our satellite clinic was a minimal operation: we shared office space and a receptionist, Lynn Olson, with Cambridge Eye Clinic.

Modern technology was a 900MHz cordless phone that could reach from the kitchen to the living room. From the ophthalmology clinic in the front of the building, Lynn could carry our cordless and, while fitting her hair dresser with brand-new frames roughly the size of safety goggles, deftly answer, "Lake Mills and Cambridge Veterinary Clinic, Lynn speaking." As if she had to clarify; Lynn knew everyone who had ever been born in town. She could expertly toggle from bending a nose pad to holding an 80-pound Labrador having anal sacs expressed.

Bean counters would eventually put numbers on what we already expected: the Cambridge branch was not profitable and it was always a stretch to staff a part-time clinic with skilled technicians. In addition, as a cat named Pumpkin and her owner would soon demonstrate, patient transfer from the satellite to the central hospital could be problematic. Eventually, CVC would sadly be shuttered like so many other businesses, but not before we would meet some life-long friends, and learn some valuable lessons.

The 9:00 a.m. Tuesday appointment on the ring-bound date book simply read, "Paula and Pumpkin, skin problems."

Paula and Pumpkin had arrived a few minutes early. I stripped from my Pella green coveralls by my truck, sloughing off remnants of the farm I had just left. As I breezed past, Lynn was wearing a not-so-subtle, "what's the rookie gonna do about this one?" smirk.

With beige linoleum floors and white cabinets, the exam room at CVC was roughly the equivalent of the kitchen from "Happy Days." In place of the inviting oval kitchen table stood a rectangular stainless steel exam table. Rather than a toaster and blender, the room sported a microscope and centrifuge.

Perched atop the exam table was Pumpkin. At this time it becomes necessary to make a confession, and clarification. I have on occasion resorted to mild exaggeration. Call it artistic license; it is an honest attempt to help more vividly build an image, and will never distract from the facts. This is not one of those occasions.

Pumpkin stood frozen in the middle of the table. She had no choice. There was no fear of her running away, and she could have fallen off the roof without a scratch. To this day, I wonder how long it had to take, because every inch of this dreadlocked domestic longhair was encrusted in matted fur.

As if it were the gold standard in feline diagnostics, I flicked Pumpkin's paralumbar fossa firmly with my middle finger. The fur was so tight she thumped like an over-ripe Georgia watermelon. Food could get in; how it got out, I have not a clue. Listening to heart sounds, feeling lymph nodes or abdominal organs would be as fruitful as a ferret in a drainpipe.

Clearly emotional, Paula stood next to the cat that she loved as her only companion. As she looked to me for help, she stroked Pumpkin's locks absently with a plastic comb, futile as a toothbrush on the hull of the USS Ronald Reagan. From her brown polyester pants and nylon jacket to the slope of her shoulders and lack of expression, it was clear that Paula was doing the best she could for Pumpkin.

Had I gone through veterinary school twice, I would have been no more prepared. I was armed with the exuberance of youth, and

 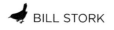 BILL STORK

had yet to spend a career's worth of compassion. I was sworn by oath to help people like Paula and cats like Pumpkin, but how

Recognizing that her needs may be well beyond the obvious, yet impossible to evaluate until she was shorn, I stalled to make a plan. We knew her teeth were bad — we could smell them. Under normal circumstances, we would take her temperature or swab something. In the absence of an available orifice, I creased my brow, stroked my chin, and "ummed" more than President Obama before Congress.

One thing was abundantly clear: this was more than even Lynn and I could handle. We needed to get Pumpkin to HQ. Recalling my near-death experience with a particular Australian Blue Heeler named Jack, I was reluctant to volunteer to transport Pumpkin.

Searching for a tone that was neither accusatory nor condescending, and attempting to camouflage my bewilderment, I folded my arms, and puffed my chest. Pointing and looking first at a random ceiling tile, I explained we would need to take Pumpkin to our main hospital. To treat her skin condition would first require finding it, and for that we would need to sedate her. The room filled with a heavy, awkward silence.

A real measure of competence in a service provider is how and if they ask your concerns. A confident doctor will face you squarely, arms extended, eyes open widely and brow raised high to connote engagement. I, on the other hand, turned half to the door, trying to escape the situation, if not the profession, as I asked "Do you have any questions?"

Pumpkin stood between us, her eyes turning from me to Paula like a small child in an inflatable sumo suit. Paula asked, "How far is it to the Lake Mills clinic?"

I answered with the first certainty of the day, "Thirteen minutes from where we stand."

Her first expression was moderate disgust. "How FAR?"

Once again failing to absorb the gravity of the situation, I responded, "Oh 'bout 11 to 14 miles, depending on whether you take A to S, or 134 to Kroghville."

Speaking in syllables so the guy with the flattop haircut and college degrees could understand, Paula asked, "What-is-the-short-est-way-from-the-Shell-sta-tion-to-your-cli-nic? And, once I get there, how close is the nearest gas station?"

Searching for simplicity and feeling a bit foolish, I volunteered to take Pumpkin to Lake Mills.

It took hours, but our ace technician Sheila was able to help Pumpkin shed the dreads. The matted fur had resulted in a Staph infection that would respond nicely to a medicated bath and antibiotics. We cleaned her teeth, her ears and trimmed her nails. We were able to make specific grooming and nutrition suggestions and, like a prisoner freed from solitary confinement, Pumpkin soon gained weight, vigor and personality.

Once Pumpkin was back in Paula's arms, I couldn't contain my curiosity, "Though it's none of my business, why did you need to know exactly how far it was to our clinic?"

"I can only go 15 miles," she answered. "I have a hole in my gas tank. If I put in more than a gallon, it pours right back out."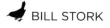

BILL STORK

Cooder

Early in the summer of 2004, Cooder struggled to his feet for what would turn out to be the last time. Down two short steps into the garage, the Dodge caravan he used for a back stop was gone for groceries. Like Bambi on ice, all four feet sprawled.

Too sore to raise his head, all I could see was the whites of his big sad brown eyes. He exhaled long and slow, "It's ok."

The last act of a legend, letting me know it was ok for him to go.

Born and orphaned in a hollowed log on the banks of the Sangamon River, he was fortunate that a kind soul in a kayak alerted the Champaign County Humane Society. His presentation to the University of Illinois Veterinary School for neuter and vaccines turned out to be a one way trip to Winfield (Vet) Village. Fourteen years, two states and a six pack of Budweiser later, he made his mark.

Apropos, as I write this story on Easter Sunday, Cooder requires no embellishment. Today, artistic license takes a break.

Cooder was always right where you needed him, never in the way. He could operate in overdrive, granny low, or comatose, as dictated by the day and time. As a 12-month-old, card-carrying Labrador Retriever puppy, whose dad was studying for National Board exams (obsessed, to say the least, with future and career riding on the outcome), Cooder slept.

During study breaks I would pull out the .38 caliber dummy launcher. The sound of the pin would set off a thundering herd including my roommate's Golden Retrievers and a mutt named Herschel. Like Rambo eluding the militia, you would never see Cooder leave. What circuitous route he must have taken is a mystery to this day. When the canvas landed 100 yards into the corn stubble and across a muddy creek, there was Cooder. He'd wait until Abby or one of the other goldens reached for it, and take off, turning the retrieval into a game of keep away.

Near graduation, my classmates and I gathered to reflect and celebrate. There was surely loud music and possibly beverage and tens of people talking about the future. At what cue we have no clue, Cooder commenced "hot laps" across the backs of 4 couches on the walls of the living room. Normally polite to a fault, of little concern were the people sitting on the couches — all of whom were weeks away from being veterinarians, and thankfully amused. Like a marble in a velodrome, he circled faster and higher. Every couple laps he would back off the throttle so Tony, the year old pit bull struggling to stay in his vapor trail, wouldn't break chase.

Cooder and I made the transition from the land of Lincoln to the land of Lombardi as best as can be expected.

By the time my central Illinois mushmouth accent would fade, my bachelor buddy was cleaning up under high chairs. Falling into a peaceful symbiosis with his "sister." my daughter Paige, on the sound of a cup of kibble dumped from a ceramic mug with his picture on it, he would come running. He would sit patiently until she said "OK."

In exchange he would absorb hugs and listen quietly when she was frustrated or mad. (A function, by the way, that continued A.D. Years later, it was not unusual to see a pensive Paige sitting next to his little wooden cross, picking at the grass and dandelions.)

Cooder evidently was not willing to risk the onset of scurvy, constipation or starvation; on one occasion consuming a half case of Valencias purchased from an FFA fund raiser. Courtesy of Cooder, there were two Thanksgivings and a Christmas when the whipped cream went solo; he had downed the pumpkin pie. DNA technology could not have proven there had ever been pie in the pan. An apologetic Labrador spent the holidays repeatedly excusing himself to the alfalfa stubble, pooping like a goose crossed with a Holstein cow.

48 compact disks in wooden crates and Rubber Maid's patented secure lock system were of little hindrance to a determined Cooder, once helping himself to 6.3 lbs of Hill's Maintenance diet in one unattended sitting. His taste for items commonly found in the "Family Planning" aisle at Walgreens is not fodder for a family publication.

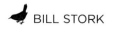 BILL STORK

He could snatch a disk flying six feet in the air, and swim as far as a PVC and hair spray cannon could shoot a tennis ball into Rock Lake. Fortunately he also had the patience of the Pope. On a Sunday evening many years ago, he lay motionless on the stainless steel surgery table with a 16-gauge needle in his neck, flowing life into a transfusion bag.

To the good fortune of a 6-year-old boy who never had the use of his legs, and the little black lab mutt, Jenny, who kept him company, Cooder's bone marrow could crank out red blood cells faster than China makes microchips.

I had just wiped my hands after checking the oil and greasing the last zerk on my lawn tractor, when the phone rang. Jenny was feeling poorly.

As I rounded the north end of Rock Lake toward the clinic, on that Sunday afternoon in 1995, the annual armada of fishermen outlined where the reeds in 36 inches of water drop to 36 feet, and spring walleye and bluegill lie in wait.

I stepped from the truck to hear the first three lawns of the year being mowed. The potpourri of last fall's yard dander and leaves in one nostril, Heidi's secret "rubbed rib-eyes" over Kingsford wafted from Keiner's grill across the yard.

Outside, Wisconsin was crawling out from under a brutal winter blanket, squeezing the last ray of daylight from the first T-shirt afternoon. Inside, secondhand cigarette smoke hung in the little yellow exam room like a Chicago blues bar on Sunday morning. Swaddled in a St. Vinnie's beach towel, Jenny lay lifeless on the stainless steel table.

Reaching for her nose from his wheelchair was Jason. She managed a thump of her tail. Angie kept her right hand on Jason's shoulder while wiping the tears with the other. Half in the door, Todd tried to be strong. A jack of all trades and a workin' man, he fidgeted looking for something to fix. Little did he know, his turn would come.

Yesterday Jenny chased balls, happy as if they'd been flung 50 yards across an empty meadow. She'd watch the ball till it stopped bouncing three squares down a concrete path, and then return it to the only spot on Jason's lap where he could flick it again.

Bloodwork confirmed what her pale gums and labored respiration suggested: Jenny had a life-threatening anemia. Why, we could only speculate, and of little clinical relevance. The only thing certain was that Jenny's survival would require blood. Doing nothing, or transport to an emergency clinic were not options. We were already well over budget. Buoyed by a young boy's hopes and a mother's tears, and compensated by the callouses in a man's hand, we called in Cooder.

Cooder weighed 72 pounds every adult day of his life, which is why we knew he had eaten exactly 6.3 lbs of kibble from the booby-trapped Rubbermaid vault, back in college. Thankfully, Jenny weighed only 58. If you will recall, medical discussions are in metric (it sounds more scientific). Dr. Stork's rough math is always in whole units, so those following at home don't have to fetch a calculator, and rounded in such a fashion that they will hold up under scrutiny.

Jenny weighed 26kg and her percentage of red blood cells was only 9%. If she were to see Monday morning, she was going to need every red blood cell Cooder had to spare.

The only spot one can hope to harvest such a volume from is the jugular vein. On command, and in character, Cooder lay still as a statue on the surgery table, 48 inches in the air. Six hundred mL of his blood drained quickly through the 16-gauge needle and heparinized tube in his neck, into the transfusion bag waiting on the floor.

Jenny lay motionless on the heating pad as the infusion pump whirred. Through the catheter in her vein, Cooder's cells became hers. She would spend three days in the hospital.

For six more years, Jenny bounced down the sidewalk to fetch the ball for Jason. 10mg of prednisone daily for the rest of her life would ensure that her immune system would not turn inexplicably against her cells again.

 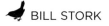 BILL STORK

That spring, Todd's payments came regular as rain. Like a trail of bread crumbs, scattered clippings and broken leaves from the riding lawn mower marked a path to the front porch, from the trailer and truck pulled in a half-circle in the parking lot.

Always near the end of the day, a cloud of two-cycle exhaust and fresh-cut grass would hang over the front counter, as Todd slipped in to leave a twenty dollar bill.

With an apology, embarrassed he had made a mess in the lobby, and a "thank you <u>sooo</u> much," he was eternally grateful to the old yellow lab named Cooder, who had saved the tears of the woman he loved, and spared the laugh of her boy and his dog.

He nodded and excused himself, as they kept supper warm for him at home. ❧

Give Me a C!

It was Saturday, December 3, 2011. There was 3:00 left on the clock and the Badgers were down by 4. Russell Wilson and the Badgers took possession inside their 20-yard line. Eight plays later, Wilson hit tight end Jacob Pedersen for a long pass play that set up Montee Ball for a Big Ten Championship 7-yard touchdown. 50,000 Badger fans at Lucas Oil Stadium, and a million more watching on TV, went wild. Meanwhile, one veterinarian tried to stay on the road.

I worked hard to focus through the double S curve just after the horse farm, as Matt Lepay called the plays like a perfectly enunciated auctioneer, pausing and growling for each completed pass and first down. His delivery became more urgent as the field got shorter and the Badgers approached history.

It can be said of many farms, but nowhere is it more true: it is an honor and a privilege to work for the Dams Dairy Farm. Matt Dams and his wife Cindy didn't put the "family" in farm, but they live it. With his parents, they farm 400 acres and milk 200 Holstein cows, just west of Columbus. In addition to receiver jars and automatic takeoffs, the milking parlor has a DVD, board games and Legos. Evening milking takes place after supper and homework, which is why I have to occasionally remind myself how much I appreciate the romance of family farms like the Dams, as it is often near midnight when I find myself winding north on State Highway 73.

"Hi, yeah, this is Matt Dams and I have a cow that started to calve around noon, and she hasn't done a thing since."

Translation: cow with a uterine torsion. As to how it might happen, a large cow carrying a small calf lunges to stand and eat. In an unfortunate "twist" of fate, the calf decides to stretch or roll at the same time. In doing so, the uterus (and the calf in it) rotates, anywhere from 90 to 270 degrees, usually clockwise. We can speculate this would render a seriously uncomfortable cow, not in the least bit able to give birth without assistance.

Faced with a twisted uterus we have three options. Third, and least favorite, is to do a Cesarean Section: surgically correcting the uter-

 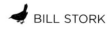 BILL STORK

us and removing the calf through the side door. Secondly, depending on topography, resources and personnel, you can leave the calf in position, and rotate the cow around her.* On this evening, my first choice was to leave the cow in place, and rotate the calf.

Lubed, scrubbed and gloved, I addressed my patient. We took a break from post-game analysis. If I could get through the birth canal, we had an excellent chance at correcting the torsion without surgery, lumber or ropes. As my arm disappeared to the shoulder, the Dams family collectively exhaled and Matt eagerly asked, "How can we help?"

Consumed with trying to assess the direction of the torsion and a prime piece of calf with which to arm wrestle, I politely asked if he could get the cow's soiled tail off my neck. Embarrassed, he quickly complied, but wasn't content to stand idly and watch.

"How about a cheer?"

As if contemplating the perfect surgical approach, I bit my bottom lip and creased my brow.

"Matt, I think that's exactly what we're gonna need."

Russell Wilson may have had 49,000 more fans, but he had nothing on Dr. Stork that day. Complete with high kicks, turns and thrusts, my four-person, Carhartt and knee boot clad squad broke into a cheer as if they had rehearsed.

"Roll the calf, roll the calf, puuuulll her out alive," they crescendoed.

With that kind of support, failure was not an option. Like a kid on a swingset getting ready to jump, I rocked the calf once, twice, and on the third I heaved as high as I could, shuffled my feet, reversed my handhold, ducked low and completed the rotation.

As the Dams family erupted in cheer, I turned my head and held my breath. Having "broken water" and relieved a 180-degree torsion, 30 gallons of fetal fluid cascaded like a viscous waterfall. A perfect wave, broken only by my neck and head, it filled my boots, splashing as it hit the barn floor.

If relieving the torsion was the touchdown, delivering a live heifer calf was the 2-point conversion. Postgame celebration was brief, as the minutes-old calf was quickly dried, dipped and fed her first quarts of colostrum.

If I practice until I'm 100, I doubt I will ever have another cheering section; a memory I will hold fondly, until the next time the phone rings at midnight, "Yeah, this is Matt Dams..."

Our second option for correcting a uterine torsion is to leave the calf where she is, and rotate the cow around her. This option is often employed when the attending veterinarian is unable to pass an arm through the cervix, or birth canal, and therefore unable to engage the calf and rotate. It may also be the method of choice when friends are visiting and you are of the mind to give them something to video with their iPhone.

Required is a long stiff rope and one fairly stout assistant not necessarily concerned about the potential of being kicked in the head. It is worthy of note that this has not happened to this practitioner. We can speculate it would not be an intentionally violent motion on the part of the patient. You also need another assistant, who surprisingly needs not be of significant physical stature. One 36" long, 2x4 inch board can increase the likelihood of success. Depending on number of, and relative strength of your assistants, a knoll, ditch or small hill can make things less labor intensive.

To start, we position our patient with a halter on her head, as if leading her into a show ring. If on a hillside, we situate her with the direction of the torsion downhill. The midpoint of our long rope is positioned over her neck, just in front of her shoulders. We cross the ropes in front of her front legs, pull them between her front legs, cross them again and pull them parallel to her ribs. We then cross the ropes over her back, parallel to her spine and crossed again over her back, just in front of her udder. Finally we drop the rope to her belly, in front of the udder, cross it one last time and extend the equal ends of rope between her back legs, handing them to the assistant with the lesser physical stature.

Behind our patient, ends of rope in hand, the first assistant watches patiently. When the cow shifts her weight in the direction of the torsion, the assistant pulls both ends of the rope equally. If all goes well, the cow will sink to the ground.

 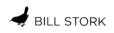 BILL STORK

Now the remaining assistants take the front and back legs and roll the expectant mother into dorsal recumbency (onto her back). Lying on her back is not natural or particularly advantageous from a selection standpoint, yet most cows in my experience seem to become fairly complacent at this point.

The lumber is laid across her belly, just cranial (in front of) her udder. If one assistant is less than 180 lbs and with low center of gravity (or a skateboarder), they mount the board. As the cow is rocked from side to side, the cow-surfing assistant applies pressure to the abdomen and therefore the calf. This pressure keeps the calf in place, as the cow is rotated in such a fashion as to relieve the twist in the uterus.

After a few cycles, the cow is rolled and righted. If you have planned well, that will be downhill. If all goes well, you have relieved the torsion and the birth canal is open. From this point, delivery is routine. Caution is exercised as often the uterus is compromised by lack of blood supply. ◈

Mary Lee

On the evening of Saturday, February 23, 2013, Mary Lee Anderson passed silently from this world. It may have be the only thing she did quietly in all her 86 years. She leaves behind many friends, her children, the Michigan Wolverines and a vet clinic. It can be said, and without a thimble of exaggeration, to her we owe our very existence.

Forty eight years ago, Dr. Robert Anderson established the Lake Mills Veterinary Clinic in his house on East Grant Street. Today we have a staff of 10, and couldn't function without anyone. In 1965, Dr. Anderson had Mary Lee.

In that time you could shoot a slingshot from any farm to the neighbors, and very few farmers treated their own cows. There were no days off or shared "on call." He practiced out of a two-wheel-drive, four door sedan, and every winter was "real." There was no emergency clinic to refer sick pets. If the phone rang, it was up to Dr. Anderson to treat the animal. Long before cell phones and GPS, it was up to Mary Lee to find him. The life of a country vet was anything but easy; without the support of Mary Lee, it would have been unthinkable. While she was veterinary technician, receptionist, accountant and cleaning staff, Mary Lee also maintained the home and was the mother of a 6-year-old and a newborn.

Mary was meticulous, and frugal to the penny. Farmers thinking they might not owe quite what their statements read would soon be shown in detail the dates, times and services rendered, as well as payments made. When men in white shirts and ties from the IRS came in search of violations, they too were shown the proper documentation. T's crossed and i's dotted, they would quickly cut a check themselves.

When the clinic moved to its current location in 1977, Mary Lee still wielded the pen and a watchful eye over the checkbook. Long before spreadsheets, and minutes after it hit the mailbox, if a drug bill exceeded $500, the phone was about to ring and there would be some 'splainin to do.

 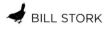 BILL STORK

The only thing more legendary than her resolve was her wit. Blessed with a nearly surgical sense of humor, she was a writer, a former editor for the New York Times, a lover of music, theater and had traveled the world. If your vision of the 60's and 70's is black, white and monotone, Mary Lee Anderson was Kodachrome and surround-sound. From NASCAR to Michigan football, and politics to current events, you would be hard pressed to find a topic she could not converse and expand upon.

When I bought the clinic in 1994, Mary Lee was gracious and supportive, if not relieved. Though she seldom ventured past her living room on Grant Street, by way of osmosis or association she seemed to always know what was taking place in the little blue clinic on Highway V. Her comments were measured, just enough that we always knew she had her finger on the pulse.

Mary, for 19 years we have practiced so as to respect what you and Dr. Anderson started, and to dignify the Veterinarian's Oath. We will do our dead level best to ensure you would be proud of where we are going. ⬦

Distracted Driver

Few young men and women have found themselves in Pella green coveralls embroidered with a Staff of Aesculapius, and black rubber boots, without having read *All Creatures Great and Small*. Having rural sensitivities and a love of animals, a trip to Val and Dave's farm should have been exactly the bait that lured you through eight years of lectures and labs.

With three kids who could walk a mile down a gravel drive in their bare feet, 65 Holstein dairy cows, and three secondhand tractors, they fed the masses. Like a living diorama at the county fair, their faded red barn sat near a winding blacktop road five miles west of Cambridge, Wisconsin, surrounded by 180 rolling acres of Irish green alfalfa, corn and soybeans.

When you drove onto the farm, either the low rumble and an intentional down-shift, or the truck tires on gravel would surely flush at least a few of the Birkrem five. If not, you were wise to give a pull on the aftermarket cow horn under the hood and find a little paperwork to do from the safety of the vehicle. At the risk of sounding like a coward, even if nobody heard you drive in, Jack did.

To put your feet on the Birkrem farm without escort was to find yourself immediately involved in an animal behavior incident with a four-year-old, intact, male Australian Blue Heeler. Herd or be herded; with 120 years of hybrid vigor and four years of daily practice, Jack was a master. Maintain a hard angle with direct eye contact and he would maintain a constant eight feet. Turn your head, or avert your eyes, and you were high-jumping onto the hood of your truck.

On this particular visit there were limping cows and coughing calves. As I scrubbed my boots and planned my next stop, Val asked what I thought of the scuff on Jack's side. The "scuff" was a large gash needing medical attention.

Thus far, I had focused on treating cattle and surviving Jack. I hadn't noticed he had a gaping 6cm gash on the right side of his chest. Let the record show that in his lifetime Jack had bounced off

 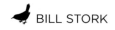

everything from a cow's foot to a FedEx truck. The only thing that cost him a day's work was a 9-iron.

So, when asked how I thought we should deal with the injury, I had to pause. My opinion had to be honest, with components of good medicine and self-preservation. There is no mention of vengeance in the Veterinarian's Oath.

My plan came immediately, but I shifted my weight, creased my brow and rearranged my John Deere hat so as to appear thoughtful.

"Wow, guys," I began, "that's a huge cut. Being on the ribs as it is, that thing will get massively infected. It would be in his best interest to anesthetize him and close it surgically."

Another pause for apparent thought, then, "You know, while he's under, it wouldn't cost a lot extra, and he would be less likely to wander off, if we were to neuter him."

Duly concerned, Val asked for an estimate of cost. My scale tipped from good business to self-preservation. If I could lower his blood testosterone from rocket fuel to diesel, I had a chance.

I anticipated that Jack had never ridden in any of the cars he had chased or bounced off. With drugs from the truck, I had a nice cocktail that would ensure 20 minutes of excellent sedation.

Regrettably, the trip to the Lake Mills Veterinary Clinic was 25 minutes.

So, with Jack safely in a drug-induced coma, resting peacefully on the passenger seat, I departed for the clinic. Warm summer breeze, window rolled down, all the while oblivious that Jack would soon be woven into the fabric of my 1990 Chevy 1500 work truck. If there was a word to describe my first veterinary service vehicle, it would be "manual." That would include both the transmission and the windows. Years before Sirius, the radio was both FM and AM

Half a decade before cell phones, I rolled along Hwy A, planning how we would transfer Jack to the clinic. Somewhere around the time I was contemplating his castration, he broke the peace like Jack Nicholson in "The Shining."

As I cautiously waited for traffic to clear at the offset intersection of Hwy 89, Jack was motionless. By the time I was northbound on Main, he had become 45 pounds of hallucinogenic heeler.

I must have dozed when my anesthesia professor William J Tranquilli (yes, really) lectured that 4-year-old Australian Blue Heelers in pickup trucks can go from surgical anesthesia to fully awake in 8 seconds.

As I shifted into second on Main Street, Jack lunged for my jugular. With a move cross-sanctioned by the AVMA and the WWF, I threw a block, pinning him against the dash. That set in motion the channel-scan function of the radio, and cranked the volume.

I'm all but certain the little blue half-ton pickup was traveling anything but a straight line.

With Jack's backside rotating past the passenger window, and the radio blasting eight seconds of everything from Cyndi Lauper to Randy Travis, we rolled. Jack was more than compliant with samples of bodily fluids: he deposited a urine sample in my King Biscuit Blues Festival coffee mug, and a fecal sample on the dashboard, heater ducts, and windshield.

I considered abandoning ship, but somehow the image of the clinic truck parked in front of the Lake Mills Golf Club with Dr. Stork on the outside and Jack gnashing and lunging inside did not seem like an image that would grow our practice. Plan B was to get the truck inside a building.

The good folks at Steve's Car and Truck Service had kept me on the road through collisions and broken fuel lines and I didn't want to wear out my welcome, but I was short on options, and losing feeling in my right hand. When I pulled up and tapped my horn, I'm not sure Sue was aware of what she was letting in.

Once inside, order was quickly restored. We were both able to bail out, retreat to our corners and settle. In the absence of stress and motion Jack calmed quickly, was moved to a crate and transported to the hospital. ❧

 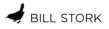 BILL STORK

Sallie

If television is a reflection of society as a whole, we've come a long way. In the '50s and '60s, Rob and Laura Petrie, and Lucy and Desi, slept in twin beds, separated by a nightstand. By the '70s, Mike and Carol Brady were still dressed in long pajama tops and bottoms, but shared a double bed. In 2014, mixed-race and same-sex couples advertise everything from Cheerios and graham crackers to Swiffers, during commercial breaks of sit-coms where characters are no longer separate, clothed or necessarily speaking the Queen's English.

I was born and raised a conservative cradle Catholic. Since the apron strings have severed, I have been impressed upon by people practicing acts of selflessness and kindness that are in no way bound by orientation or ethnicity. I've come to define the family as a group of people loving without condition, mutually respectful and universally supportive.

Which is not to say the traditional family has gone extinct. As proof I present Don, Becky, Brett and Aaron.

Brett and Aaron are the boys who hold the door, tuck their shirts and never miss a please and thank you. They show respect for their elders, as demonstrated by Mr. and Mrs., and answer the phone, "Good evening, Wilson residence."

The boys are reflective of a mother who clerked at the local bank, but was the second grade home-room mother who always had a plate of brownies. She used her vacation days to chaperone field trips to the Shedd Aquarium and Vilas Zoo, with sack lunches in big yellow buses.

Don was a free-lance handyman with a half-ton pickup and a ladder rack. He never turned down or was late for a job, parent-teacher conference or the Swing Choir Christmas concert. Luxuries were subtle and few, and paid for by after-hours cash projects: painting farm scenes on big black rural mailboxes, or building trailer hitches and additions for neighbors' pontoon boats. After bedtime stories were read, and boys were tucked in.

Following the boys home from their bus stop was to learn that first impressions and book-cover judgments need to go the way of the K-Car. At the last stop on a dead-end road, you'll find a picket fence that even Tom and Huck could never have resurrected, held up more by volunteer day-lilies, Queen Anne's Lace and burdock than the rotten posts. One corner of the gate hangs from the rotten wood, and the other rests in the mud. The house is flanked by rusted wheel barrows and mowers robbed of a carburetor and plastic fuel tank, rather than landscape timbers, bagged red cedar mulch from Menards, and hostas.

Waiting for them, bound by loyalty rather than physical restraint, was Sallie. Five years old the day Brett started High School, Sallie was a Cocker Spaniel cross with the demeanor of an old nanny who had evolved in the likeness of her family.

N7787 Clearview Road would have fit more on the gravel path between Tunica and Tutwiler, Mississippi, than a country blacktop in Dodge County, Wisconsin. Yet no Wilson ever shied or apologized.

The first sign was the faded red bandana molded to Becky's head, tied tightly behind her ears. Then the flesh slowly melted and color faded from her cheeks. At first they strained and eventually trembled, but her lips never failed to form a smile. She would never miss the boys' football game, but huddled under hood and blanket from the season opener in mid-September. Mother Teresa must have known Becky Wilson when she said, "Blessed are the sick." Proving to her boys that you will never lose if you always fight, the tumors that ravaged her abdomen could not touch her soul.

By the time Aaron started seventh grade, the boys no longer had field trips to chaperone or brownies to bake for the sale. Becky was too weakened to greet the customers at the bank. On Becky's insistence, the boys would never miss practice. On Don's orders they would hurry home.

Don worked every minute he had to keep the corrugated tin roof over their heads. Sallie could not fetch a blanket, pour tea or blunt the pain, but she never left Becky's side.

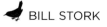 BILL STORK

Cars parked bumper-to-bumper, angled half in the ditch, lined the dead-end road. Friends, family and neighbors filed out. Everyone parted with a handshake-hug and carefully enunciated, "A-N-Y-T-H-I-N-G you need...." knowing they were going home to their life and family still intact.

What the Wilson men needed most, Becky had shown them every day of her 42 years. For the three years Becky battled, the Wilsons were a family fighting cancer. When the last glass casserole was returned, they were on their own.

Brett graduated from high school, helped his dad with big jobs and went to Madison Area Technical College in their diesel mechanic program. Aaron got straight As, played running back, fullback and catcher. Don devoted every ATP to his boys, either providing for or spending time, ensuring they were the men Becky would expect them to be.

Sallie's annual veterinary visits became every 6 months, and eventually even more frequent. It was never spoken but when her time came, the Wilsons would lose their mother all over again.

I made no attempt to hold back the flood when I knelt to feel Sallie's lymph nodes. Tears pooled in the rim of my glasses. A gentleman in jeans, Don spoke so I didn't have to.

"Doc, I'd like to take her home so the boys and I can spend one last night." I shook his right hand with a full-on shoulder clasp without raising my head. He pulled his hood, cradled what was left of the little cocker and faded into the drifting snow.

Two years later, in the second half of Aaron's last night of high school football, I leaned on the chainlink next to Don. He had walked the 50-yard line and received the bouquet players give to their mothers on "senior night."

Without taking his eyes off the game, in a tone barely audible he told me about Sallie's last night. They had shared a last supper and all gone to bed. Sallie slept on a pad in the kitchen; she wasn't able to go any farther. At 3:15 a.m. the entire house was awakened by her bark.

When the boys tried to walk, they found themselves dazed and nauseous. They fought through the carbon monoxide fumes to find Sallie sitting and staring at the old gas stove. In the howling January wind the pilot light had blown out.

Living in the hearts of those they left behind, Becky... and Sallie are a light that will never so much as flicker.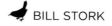

The Boutros Brothers

I was recently asked to speak to Mrs. Haviland's Health Professions class at Lake Mills High School. Sue and her miniature dachshund, Ilse, are among our favorite people and pets at the clinic. My son is a freshman and my daughter is a junior, so I thought it might be an excellent opportunity to get a peek into their world. Ask a high school kid how their day was, and if you're lucky you get a monosyllabic grunt.

Being genuinely proud of my profession, our clinic, Lake Mills and all wrapped up in this folksy veterinarian-writer persona, I could not wait. With the help of my son, I prepared my very first "Power-Point" presentation. I consider myself realistic, but with a high-tech presentation that started with the Staff of Aesculapius displayed on a 4 foot screen, how could they not be stomping, clapping and waving the lights of the cell phones in unison when I finished with the all-inclusive wisdom of the Web Wilder Credo?

I had a vision of walking out of the classroom with 13 new followers of our blog, and not a business card left in my pocket. As it turned out, I was able to keep nine of twelve mostly awake for 40 minutes, and was eternally grateful that school regulations prohibit texting during class.

The obligatory question in any such presentation is, "how did you become interested in (insert profession)?"

At this point you face the class squarely and pause. You drop your head and voice, crease your brow and stroke your chin.

"Well kids, when I was even younger than you, I had a collie dog named Sugar, and we had a vet named Dr. Van Alstine..."

What I did not tell them, is that what got me through school and has allowed me to survive 21 years of practice is not so much my keen analytical mind.

It is my ability to sleep.

With a tip of my John Deere cap to my dad, the ability to sleep anywhere, under any circumstances, is some part genetic and to some extent learned. As with most things, it is perfected and adapted to your particular profession, situation and life-style. Nothing makes one appreciate a good night's sleep like knowing when you lie down that you have an excellent chance of having to spring from bed and ear tag 150 calves.

My first day at the Lake Mills Veterinary Clinic was June 15, 1992. Somewhere in the hand-shake contract between the old school Purdue graduate and the rookie, I missed the clause about emergencies. As it turned out, it is simply "understood" that while on call, you live in town. This was a bit awkward, as I had already set up my stereo and paid a damage deposit on a farm house on a beautiful rolling drumlin on Switzke Road, just east of 'Crick.

Not only was I squarely in the geographic center of our practice area, but I could be to the clinic in 8 minutes. Unfortunately, the extra 5 minutes could mean the difference between life and death. Though the nice lady at the phone company assured me the clinic phone could be forwarded to a "699" number just as easily as a "648." Dr. Anderson knew otherwise. In 1992 cell phones were in their infancy, and they were hard wired into the dash of your truck. Being on call meant staying within earshot of a land-line. If you needed to mow grass, you had to hop off the tractor and check the answering machine every couple rounds.

Dr. Anderson was a former military man defined by his German persistence. Not to mention, he signed my paycheck. So we reached a compromise: for $80 a month, I found a bed 6 blocks from HQ for my every third night on call. Imagine being a 28-year-old recently graduated veterinarian, renting a room in an assisted living facility. Left to do over again, I may have been more charmed and made an attempt to get to know my octogenarian roommates, and probably had great stories to write about them. As it were, I snuck in, slept, and got out as fast as I could.

Back to the calves needing ear tags... Don and Larry Boutros were among the nicest folks you could ever meet. They were always polite, and even brought Arthur Bryant's Barbecue from Kansas City. They hailed from southern Missouri, and based on their drawl and

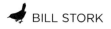 BILL STORK

demeanor, their home must have been not too awful far from the Kentucky border.

The Boutros were order buyers. They traveled throughout Wisconsin on Mondays, buying Holstein calves, and then delivered them to producers in the South and West. The last stop out of Wisconsin was Equity Livestock Auction in Johnson Creek. In order to track the movement of the animals, they required identification and documentation.

To keep the brothers rollin' and get the calves to their next meal, the goal was to move through Equity as efficiently as possible.

Their travels were dictated by the markets. Long before GPS and cell phones, we had no way of knowing if they would be calling just before the late local news, or 20 minutes before CNN came back on the air. Some Mondays, they did not come at all.

It can be said that anyone's greatest strength, can at times be their weakness. So, at 2:15 a.m. one Tuesday I sat bolt upright in bed, trembling. The Boutros Brothers had called, and I had fallen back asleep. Long before cell phones and call logs, I had no way of knowing whether 10 minutes or two hours had passed, so I dove into my Pella green coveralls and tore out in a streak. My powder blue Chevy "WT" was a half-ton 6-cylinder, but she had snort.

I slid into the gravel lot, scrambling the drugs in my vet box like Bo and Luke in the General Lee. In my rear view I saw a 1-ton diesel with a 35-foot stock trailer and Missouri plates.

Convinced they had waited for hours, I pulled alongside and stuck my head out the window, inhaling to launch my apology.

Before I could say a word, Don drawled, "W' hey Dawk, what're you doin' here? We just had a bite t'eat up at the Pine Cone and was fixing to give y'all a call, and here you is!" &

Bambi

Though the judge was kind, she stood dead last in her class at the Jefferson County Fair. She presented well, her condition was good, but her conformation left much to be desired: a bit post-legged, and not necessarily symmetrical.

Always gracious, and never one to beg favors, my daughter nodded politely and smiled. If the judge only knew...

There was no blue ribbon, but victory is not always defined by trophies and titles. Were it not for the tenacity of a young girl, the will of a stubborn little Jersey and a bit of divine intervention, she would never have stood at all.

The first call of the day was one you hope to never hear. A cow had calved the night before. As mom stood to lick and allow her to nurse, she stepped on her right rear leg.

The fracture was complete and the prognosis was poor; the decision was made to put her down. I walked at a glacial pace to the truck and back. Avoiding her big brown eyes, I placed the needle in her vein and raised my thumb to end her pain. Then pulled it back out.

The cost to treat a calf with a shattered femur is prohibitive to a farm. The chance to save a life is beyond measure, for a father and his daughter. Until we knew her final fate, Paige chose not to name her. Three months, six radiographs and five casts later, we helped her up and she staggered across the yard. With time she gained strength, and learned to use all four legs.

When asked how I know there is a God, I will often answer... Bambi. ☙

   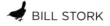 BILL STORK

Those Who Have the Least...

It is said that a business evolves in the image of its owner. In one particular sense, I regret to report that is absolutely the case. I have no excuse. My mother's kitchen was spotless. The Tupperware and pans were arranged large to small, and you never had to search for a lid. On the wall in my dad's garage hung wrenches 3/8 to 1-1/4 on nails in a perfect arch. Every screwdriver had a holster from small to large; flat-blade, Phillips and Torque

Starting with a legendary maroon tri-fold ring binder that held every paper from 8th grade to present day, I have struggled to achieve organization. At every turn, I have failed miserably. Skilled people with the best of intentions and degrees in accounting have tried. I have had phone in hand and as many as 9 of 10 digits dialed; fully intent on calling the professionals in Madison at "Ducks in a Row." Each time I cringe and hang up, fearful that in the end they will run for their cars gnashing and cursing.

And so it goes for the blue countertop in our pharmacy. Flying squarely in the face of the notion that "our level of organization speaks to the quality of our care," the catastrophe is clearly visible each time the pocket door lurches open and clients in the exam rooms see into the pharmacy.

From east to west, there is a Fred Flintstone model Dell workstation computer, flanked with a horizontal file that Claire has prepared with the forms we use most frequently. The forms are absolutely organized, but hidden from view by Mt. Clark: anointed with Starbucks dark roast and jicama splatter, Dr. Clark's pile of client records sits in various stages of development. By her nature thorough, she leaves not a single cell unturned. Near the peak is the file for the pup she saw yesterday; closer to the base is the case she's worked on since her Subaru was new.

Continuing our journey philosophically and geographically from "left" to right, we find an 8x10.5 slot so that Dr. Stork can rest a record if he has to dash into the 3:30, by 3:40. Next is the not-so-compact or accurately named "fastest and most silent printer on the market," next to another of Steve Job's museum pieces. Somewhere behind is a couple of power strips, certified code, and a blood tube stand.

Ask any of us, and I guarantee we would first deny what we would be forced to confess: any time past 8:00 a.m., like ten of Pavlov's pups, every time we pass the counter we are looking and hoping for a treat wedged between the clutter or precarious atop Mt. Clark.

Near Christmas we look and hope for Kate Dahl's mountain of goodies. Any time after noon on a summer day, we're hoping Mittsy has made a batch of vanilla and coffee frozen custard. Late June to early July, we're trolling for one of Sheila's strawberry tortes. Any one of the above will loosen your belt and lift your spirits for the rest of the day.

Five years ago I looked to the counter, and stopped dead in my tracks. Just to the left of the antique Dell sat two packs of Dollar Store "cream" filled sandwich cookies. The smile has yet to leave my face; the lesson will last forever...

In excess of 80 years old, opaque, round glasses precarious on his bulbous nose as cloudy as the mature cataracts in both eyes, William Wegner shuffled into our clinic. We waited for him to push them up, else they fall to the floor. Pre-osteoporosis he may have stood 5'6." He wore a pair of St. Vinnie's khakis that last belonged to a power-forward, gathered over shoes and laces none of which matched, and yesterday's grape jelly. One shirt tail out, the other stuffed into the belt that gathered the britches, he was a dead ringer for Quincy Magoo, minus the polish. How he found his way from Waterloo, I have not a clue.

Towing him through the door were Millie and Jasper. Each moved by rocking themselves first to one side and then the other. Technically a cross between a Shih Tzu and a Dorset lamb, they were roughly the size of an over-sized carry-on piece of luggage. If they were to find themselves standing and high centered, their paws would barely touch the ground.

Arriving without an appointment, he stood in the center of the lobby. His surroundings but a blur, Mr. Wegner stared straight ahead,

 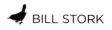

waiting for a greeting to orient him. Rightly assuming his hearing was little better than his sight, Claire shouted, "Good afternoon, sir, can we help you?"

As it turned out, we could, and he is a prime reason why I love my staff and profession.

For many years, Mr. Wegner was a landlord in Milwaukee. I'm going to extrapolate that he did not manage properties on the lakefront or in the arts district. By way of clear injustice — in his mind — he had spent the last 7 years in jail.

His nearest family of any sort was in Jefferson County, where he found an abandoned trailer home. For two Wisconsin winters, Millie and Jasper were his only companionship and source of heat.

I've only allowed the thought to pass briefly and exorcised it quickly from my head: if we were to have met Mr. Wegner 30 years previous, or been one of his tenants, our sympathy may have not run so deep. As for today, across the exam table sat an old man in need.

Millie and Jasper were infested with fleas. Their fur was matted to the open sores over their backs and chest. In a semi-circle where each of their little legs could scratch, they were raw and bald. M and J were as giddy as he was surly, so long as there was a steady cadence to the delivery of freeze-dried liver.

Conserving his meager resources, we dug deep into historic remedies and Dr. Clark's drawer of repurposed pharmaceuticals (donated by kind clients whose pets had passed, or no longer needed the medications). In weeks we had their skin calmed very nicely.

In months and a few years to follow, under Dr. Clark's guidance, the weight would come down from that of a small ruminant, to a body condition score only a bit in excess. Like a home town hound version of the "Biggest Loser," he would stop twice a month for a weight check. More often if he were lonely.

When he did, whether there was time or not, either Claire or Megan would sit for a bit. They'd encourage him for the fabulous job in taking the weight off the kids, or just ask how he was, then listen.

Mr. Wegner has since passed. On one such visit, he inverted the pockets of the same khakis and dug through his loose change and small bills to make a payment.

And from the crumpled plastic bag that hung from his wrist, he produced those two small packs of cookies. ⬦

 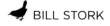 BILL STORK

Dingleberry Moments

Five years ago, 9017 Hwy 18, Cambridge, Wisconsin, became re-classified from a single-family dwelling, to a zoo. Peacefully co-existing on a seven-acre postage stamp that has come to be named "Stork Valley," there live a constant rotation of Wyoming work horses, a rescued Clydesdale who loves to eat treats from walking neighbors, and a part time barrel racing paint named Santana.

There is a pride of the best kept barn and garage cats, who have been conditioned to "sleep with one eye open," lest they be attacked by a young grey cat aptly named "Stinker" (aka Farm Dog). Any-where from two to four Alpine goats keep the scrub brush trimmed high enough to mow under with a tractor and brush hog. (I don't own a brush hog, but if I did I could get under the trees on the trac-tor and it sounds really manly.) They also get really excited at the sight of a stainless mixing bowl, and make funny squishy noises when a cute redhead feeds them kitchen scraps.

Token is a 5-year-old heeler cross who is in charge of ensuring no squirrel or chippy touches the grass, and no groundhog shows their whiskers. To my amazing fortune, this flock came as a package deal, in two loads on a 3-slot horse trailer, behind a 1-ton Ford du-ally.

Somewhere shortly before, and often after, sunset as the only ac-ceptable antidote for 12 hours of middle- managing 30 horse-lov-ing medical professionals, she sashays into her sanctuary. Malls and bars of little concern, she is at home with her herd. Trotting on her left and tapping the back of her empty hand with a cold dry nose is an eleven-year-old legendary lab named Remmi. For the rest of the evening, like a traffic cone next to a Wisconsin Electric bucket truck, Remmi will sit quiet and attentive, marking her place on the farm.

As tranquil as the Dalai Lama, the two things that will raise Rem-mi's pulse (that are not tennis balls and shotguns) are thunder-storms over Grant and Iowa Counties, and harsh words. She can sleep sound as a soldier through a hurricane just outside the bed-room window, but as the storm approaches west of Madison, she is pacing and panting. Let fly with ten decibels more angst than a Sunday afternoon matinee of James Taylor's Greatest Hits, and Rem will first attempt to mediate. If that fails, she will quickly evacuate.

Two traits that define Sheila Barnes are accountability and calm. Conflict anywhere within her sphere is for her to have failed. For the sake of clarity, her sphere is defined as anywhere within eyesight, earshot, or a half-day's drive from anywhere she has been, or plans to go in the next six months. Resolving is not good enough. It should have been anticipated and prevented, without the owners knowing "it" ever existed. Like a gate agent facing a three hour delay and a full flight, she is the calm before, after, and during the teeth of the storm.

There are exceptions to every rule. Imagine, if you will, a Friday afternoon when my dad has come to visit. Kind enough to help fix some things at the clinic, he arrives at home a few minutes before Sheila and I. A veteran of the construction unit of the US Navy, and a 50-year career sitting at the clutch and throttle of 250-ton tower cranes powered by screaming Detroit Diesels, decades before OSHA required sound guards and ear protection, the old guy doesn't hear too well.

Speaking loudly enough to hear himself, he stops to greet Remmi. Unfamiliar, and to her sounding like the famous "Mad Ref" on Monday Night Football, Remmi heads for safety. Which happens to be eight miles down Hwy 18, at the home farm.

When a dog known as a shadow goes missing, the wheels fall off.

Thankfully there is no shortage of kindness in the world. A nice lady noticed an older dog trotting down the ditch, and gave her a ride to the Humane Society of Jefferson County. In an hour and a flurry that Dr. Stork is not particularly proud of, Rem was returned to the safety of home.

That one episode of going AWOL was the most collective drama Remmi had provided in her entire life. She is most content in the back seat of any vehicle that moves, napping. As coincidence would have it, that was right where she was, and what she was supposed to be doing when Ryan Haack called for a calving problem. Young,

 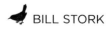 BILL STORK

strong, experienced and skilled, if Ryan calls for a calving, you have work to do.

Out of respect for Trek execs and having used my "get out of jail free" card from Chief Delaney, I eased around the north end of Rock Lake at a scant "5(to 10) over." As the road went wide and town faded in the rear view, I throttled up.

As I did, from the back seat where Remmi and Token standardly sleep, there came quite a clatter. Focusing on the road, it was neither safe nor prudent to turn and see what was the matter. As fate would have it, that would not be needed.

It was that time in spring when the grass has just turned Ireland green. Remmi, Token and every other able dog on the planet spend 10 days to two weeks doing their best imitations of small ruminants. Equipped with teeth designed to tear flesh rather than shear and grind grass, and one simple stomach rather than four, means that lush green grass has a tendency to pass... untouched and intact.

While I was embroiled in thought as to how I might extract the calf, like Timmy down the well, Rem poked my elbow with her nose and panted. Not pleased with my distraction, she mounted the spacious center console where more often rests a clipboard, or a bowl of leftover chili.

In a fashion that would be considered most atypical even in the front yard, she commenced doing pirouettes. By her third rotation, centrifugal force and my keen sense of observation made for a slam-dunk diagnosis...

Clinging to a strand of Timothy grass that may have been anchored in her transverse colon, were three Milk Dud-sized increments of excrement.

We strictly forbid our kids from texting and driving. Just to the south, Illinois has outlawed the use of cell phones on the road. I can only imagine the legal consequences of driving during the distraction of a "Dingleberry Moment."

I shouldered the rig and grabbed a glove. Quicker than a Matt Kenseth pit stop at Daytona, we were westbound and down. By the time I filled my bucket at the Haack farm, Rem was sound asleep in the back seat. ◆

BILL STORK

A Dog Called Boy

Mother Teresa said, "Blessed are the Sick." It has taken me a solid decade, and the acquaintance of a 6-year-old Doberman and his family, to absorb the beauty in that statement.

One morning, Boy was a bit slow to get up and eat his breakfast. When his family came home that afternoon, his face was swollen and his lymph nodes were the size of tennis balls. My heart sank when I took the call, and the staff fell silent as he approached the clinic. It did not take long to confirm the diagnosis that we suspected, Lymphosarcoma.

What took place in the year that followed was a demonstration of all that is beautiful in the human- animal bond. Boy's family did not hesitate. Within days he was being treated at the UW Veterinary School, and within months was in remission.

Thanks to the expertise of the Vet School, the unconditional love of his family, and the untouchable spirit of Boy, he lived his last year much like his first five.

Through it all, Boy was charming, cooperative and energetic. Thanks to him and his family, we have relearned the age old lessons of never giving up and enjoying every day.

Boy lived every quality day he had, and if he suffered, he didn't let it show.

Take Notes, Kim Kardashian

72-day, $20 million weddings may be good for the Kardashians. Speaking for myself, I'm looking to keep up with Robbie the farm hand.

Einstein's Theory of General Relativity states that: *Quantities measured are relative to the observer's velocity, excepting the speed of light.* For example, the faster Eddie Lacy is able to run while carrying a football, the more money he will find on his debit card.

Ryan Haack's Theory of Relativity (HTR) dictates that: *The anticipation of cold is often relatively more painful than the experience.* Variables in the HTR include wind speed and direction as well as the facilities you have to work in. The intricacy/grunt ratio and duration of the procedure are crucial factors.

Speaking purely in the hypothetical, Mark and Dorothy (honey and sweetie) Christenson have a recently fresh (just had a baby) heifer with a prolapsed uterus. Let's say she doesn't care for the Christmas music on the country station so she crawls onto the snowpack of the dooryard, dragging 185 lbs of recently vacated uterus behind. Let's say there is a veterinarian (bare-chested as they often are) attempting to restore that uterus to a more sustainable anatomic position. It is not a procedure that requires the precision of assembling microchips. Some combination of the oration and the physical output is going to ensure that when you stand in victory you'll be shrouded in steam like a Gatorade commercial, regardless of what your dashboard computer says the temperature is.

Then there is barnyard surgery. Farmers work hard to ensure their cows, expectant mothers in particular, have the ultimate in cow comfort, feed availability and friendly roommates. In the face of our best efforts, giving birth to a baby the size of an eighth grader will occasionally come to involve stress. Her intake, digestion and fermentation will be interrupted and she may displace the last of her four stomachs (the abomasum). Options are to leave the abomasum where it is, and rotate the cow around it, or surgically correct it.

While right-flank abomaso-omentopexy may sound as technically

BILL STORK

challenging as pre-frontal lobotomy... brain surgery it ain't. Suture material may be the size of deep-sea fishing line and instruments may say Snap-On. Pexies also don't take place in a climate-controlled suite by surgeons in scrubs and gowns with nurses to wipe their brow and hand them instruments. On a good day, we have a custom-designed breakaway surgery stall with padded floor, lights and an LB White propane space heater blowing on our back.

Cows may displace the day after New Year's on the Weichmann farm. The wind-chill in Dean's holding area (surgical suite) is an obligatory 10-%15 higher than the front door of a Catholic Church on top of a hill. The prevailing northwest wind is accelerated as it funnels from Minot, North Dakota, through the cracks between his free stall and barn. Surgical gowns have a tendency to drag in the cow manure, so the site is kept clean by the surgeon stripping to the waist and gloving to the pit. If a veterinarian finds himself doing back to back surgeries, his or her hands may be in danger of falling right off the end of his arms. In such cases, the reality of the cold has surpassed the anticipation (dread), and therefore inverted the HTR.

Then there is the Stork Corollary to the Haack Theory of Relativity, which states: *There are times when the experience of an acquaintance defies the elements.* You find yourself driving away with your core warmed like a hearthstone.

It was a Christmas, I have not a clue the year. The day we celebrate the birth of Jesus as it were, it was not to be attempted without SmartWool, polypropylene, fleece and Gore-Tex. Insulated coveralls sealed the bottom and top, and a balaclava topped with your thickest Carhartt tuque finished off the ensemble. You triaged and assembled your instruments and medications in the attached garage. Bare-hand budget and face time were at an all-time low.

Three hundred thousand into its half-million mile career, the '94 Cummins diesel started in the garage; we would not take a chance by shutting her off. With all due respect to the environmentalists in the crowd, you tucked the truck behind the parlor, made sure the heater was on "blast furnace" and let it run. There was no guarantee the fuel would not gel and you were for certain going to need every BTU you could buy in 30 minutes.

Robbie met me at the truck, removed his glove and shook my hand. As he let my heels back to the ground, he clasped my shoulder, wished me a "Merry Christmas," and thanked me for coming out as if I had a choice over obligation. He didn't mention, and his demeanor never acknowledged, the ongoing polar vortex.

There were four chained gates between the truck and the cow. A 1200 lb Holstein will make Harry Houdini look like a kindergarten card-trick novelty when it comes to escaping. I toted my bucket and rope while Robbie led the way, repeatedly stuffing gloves in his armpit to unwind, unchain and latch, and sink precious heat from his hands to the galvanized steel gates. I hunched my shoulders to maintain the seal between collar and cap.

Most farmers would make idle talk about the weather or none at all. Robbie asked where I was from, where I went to school and what my parents did for a living. The cow had managed to crawl forward in the sand stall. Robbie wedged himself between the brisket bar and clavicle of the cow and heaved. At the same time I pulled, and in 3 harmonious hunches we had her comfortable. I set my gloves on the cow's rump while I knelt to set the needle in her vein. Just as quickly Robbie picked them up and stuffed them in his pocket, far more concerned about my comfort, than his.

As calcium ran into the cow, I learned Robbie had worked on this farm for three years. He spoke of the farm and herd in personal pronouns and terms of endearment, ownership, and pride. He had graduated from school nearby and his parents had worked on a local farm for most of their 25-year marriage.

As the bottle drained and the cow came back to life, he excused himself without walking away. In a manner neither apologetic nor pretentious, he called his girl to apologize that he was going to be a few minutes longer. He told her he was looking forward to sharing Christmas dinner with her, could not wait to give her a present, and that he loved her.

On a frigid Christmas day, I got a beautiful lesson in respect, accountability, loyalty and unpretentious love, courtesy of a 22-year-old, second generation farmhand. ❧

 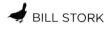 BILL STORK

Angler of the Year

Slim-Fast, Weight Watchers and Dr. Atkins have nothing on Tricks and Minnie.

Tricks is an 18 lb Jack Russell Terrorist. Minnie is her nearly cylindrical dachshund sidekick.

In addition to proper vaccination, heartworm and parasite prevention, a physical exam is of vital importance for the health and well-being of your pet. Our physical starts when you get out of the car. We are observing their pace and energy, looking for lameness and skin conditions, observing for head shaking or rubbing. We pore through the history for existing conditions.

We greet the guys with freeze-dried liver, and then we ask questions about lifestyle, diet and exercise.

In such an exam with one of our favorite clients, and two of our favorite patients, I asked, "What do they eat?"

She answered, "Mostly bullheads, some catfish, and bluegill on special occasions."

You see, Tricks and Minnie have a pond. Each morning, Tricks becomes an 18 lb Jack Russell missile, straight into the water. She circles, dives, and surfaces with a fish, then swims to shore and places it at the feet of her grateful friend Minnie, the dapple-grey Dachshund, who is evidently less of a fisherman.

Tricks repeats the process until she figures Minnie has enough; then continues until she's caught her meal, all the while abiding by Wisconsin size and bag limits. She requires no license as she is well under 16.

For the life of me, I can't find fault in their self-imposed diet plan. It's the ultimate in low-carb, balanced, organic, green, local, and sustainable.

Rip

When author Michael Perry is asked where he finds inspiration to write, his answer is "John." John occupies the corner office of the New Auburn bank, and holds his home mortgage.

If asked where I find motivation to continue to practice, my answer would be... "Rip." The double entendre has never been more appropriate.

Rip was the happiest dog on the planet. He was a 60 lb yellow lab with a 10 lb tongue, and he was not afraid to use it. To know Rip, was to be licked and loved.

The maples will never turn yellow, red and orange that I don't think of Rip. It was this time of year when he was running happily in his yard on a windy fall day. From nowhere appeared a stray plastic bag that blew over his head, spooking him to the point that he ran headfirst and full speed into a tree.

As fate would have it, Rip's owner was a veterinary technician at the Lake Mills Veterinary Clinic. Though he did not move or respond, radiographs could find no fractures, and blood work confirmed that his organs continued to function.

We all took turns supporting him day and night with fluids, nutrition and preventing bedsores and pulmonary congestion. On any given day, it is safe to say that either Rip's owner, or I, were ready to give up. Rip never did.

After three weeks he was able to lift his head. Nearly a month after having T-boned a tree, to cheers and tears from the staff, he was able to walk.

Although his navigation and balance remained less than perfect, in time Rip was back to licking and loving everyone in sight.

Thanks to Rip, when presented with a pet sick or injured, we will never stop trying. ❧

 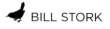

Buck

In 1844, Norwegian immigrants built twin Lutheran Churches at the top of one of the most beautiful rolling hills in southern Wisconsin, separated by 50 paces and belief in predestination. In the shadow of those twin steeples, on a chair sits Dan, his head against the tobacco shed behind him.

His gloved right hand rests on a Browning 20 gauge over and under, his left hand on Buck's expansive head. A quarter inch of frost diffracts the rising October sun into every color from amber to magenta, on a morning so still the grazing cows look like statues. The only movement is from untouched tears meandering through the cracks in Dan's face, and the slow rise and fall of Buck's chest, as he takes his last few breaths.

45-year-old construction workers don't choose to live in apartments above their buddy's garage, and there was never mention of child or wife. Likely his closest family was lying on a flannel blanket between his camo boots, as he had for the last 12 years. In six weeks cancer had taken his strength and stamina, his spirit untouched.

Not a word was spoken as I lay in the gravel to give the final injection. I stood to walk away and the silence was broken by the Browning. Dan fired two final shots over his friend and Buck took his last breath. Two grown men in Carhartts and coveralls were left standing, crying in a barnyard, officially laying waste to the old notion about first impressions.

The compassion of our staff was in overdrive the day Buck first followed Dan into a veterinary clinic. His head was carried low, left rear leg dangling, eyes on Dan.

Oblivious to the hours posted and that the clinic was dark, Dan bellied up to the counter and announced the obvious, "Somethin's wrong with ma dog." Because it's who they are, and no one with a pulse could deny the devotion in that dog's eyes, our people activated. Meticulous by nature, with a keen interest in sports medicine, Dr. Clark examined Buck.

The diagnosis was more obvious than how to tell Dan. Buck had torn several ligaments and the meniscus in his knee. It would require significant surgery if he were ever to retrieve another bird.

At times like these we look to the owner's response. There was none. Fifteen minutes later, Buck limped and Dan staggered back to their ten-year-old F150 with a two-week supply of pain medication.

As the door shut behind them, in their void was a fog of second-hand smoke and four heavy hearts. All of us were certain that Buck's remaining years would be bound to a couch, and painful.

Ten days later, Dan returned. With Buck still in tow, purpose in his stride, and far more likely to pass a field sobriety test, he laid a wad of cash on the counter that startled Frida to the safety of the pharmacy. Without counting, I wasn't sure whether he wanted us to treat his dog, or buy the place, until he asked, "Where do we start?"

He didn't seem to notice the pause, as we all stood looking slack-jawed.

We tested Buck for heartworm and Lyme disease, dewormed and vaccinated him. We scheduled surgery with Dr. Laing two weeks later. The damage was as extensive as Dr. Clark had diagnosed. There were weeks of recovery, rest and pain management.

To follow were weeks of rehabilitation, all of which Dan followed to the letter.

By the time the frost fell and leaves turned, Buck was back out front, pointing, flushing and retrieving. Head held high, eyes on Dan.

As I lay on the floor like a mechanic in a white lab coat, removing the skin staples, I felt for the right time and asked, "Dan, it's none of my business, but where'd you come up with that money?"

He shrugged, quick and nonchalant. "Jus' sold my Harley."

Never again would we let a first impression judge a man, or doubt his devotion to his dog.

 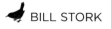 BILL STORK

All Gave Some

I can't imagine a more spectacular place than southern Wisconsin in May. Rust red hip-roof dairy barns are wrapped in Ireland green pastures of alfalfa, with herds of black and white Holsteins ambling about as they have for three generations. Others are but monuments to tradition, tenacity and productivity. Fence lines and lane ways are flanked by dogwoods and lilacs in all their glory.

Plan to be at least distracted, or just pull over and take a picture for the wallpaper on your cell phone. Use all your given senses and go slowly. Close your mouth and gently pull the country air through your nostrils. Taste the loam, peat and sand of a freshly worked field. Chisel-plowed in fall, disked, dragged, picked clean of stones, and finished during five straight God-given days of dry just last week.

Deep horizontal lugs on tractor tires form perfect arcs at the headlands, giving way to parallel lines that merge to the horizon. Seed lies an inch below the soil. With a lot of hope, a little prayer and some rain, it will become feed and forage in October when the south winds shift north and crisp.

A bike ride or drive down a country road can be an event unto itself; pure sensory overload, no i-pod, widescreen or digital enhancement.

Unless you are Jason Stevens*. For him, it is horrifying.

We have known Jason, his wife and their pets for the better part of a decade. It could be the camo fatigues, sewn name badge, and a calico cat named HumVee, but I had always suspected a military background, despite the fact that even in uniform he looks as dangerous as the assistant manager at Kwik Trip.

In a recent visit, HumVee was not always using his litter box. While our technicians analyzed a sample, we had time to talk. As it turns out, he is a veteran of six tours of duty between Iraq and Afghanistan. His job is a combat medic. Jason stopped short of any details, but while he was out of the room his wife explained. He would be dropped from a helicopter on a giant lead weight called a "canopy buster." On the ground, he often had to fight hand-to-hand with knives and sidearms just to get to a fallen soldier he hoped to save.

When he returned, I was trying to put things into perspective. I asked, "What's the hardest thing about being stateside?"

"Driving," was his instant answer.

As I stood slack-jawed and silent, he explained. A McDonald's bag blown from the bed of a pickup is a potential roadside bomb, ready to detonate and destroy a passing convoy, and mangle the soldiers on a mission. The bridge over the Rock River or the underpass at Hwy N? Perfect places for an ambush.

Over the next few days, I noticed all of the roadside litter I drive past every day, and each underpass I blithely roll beneath. Still trying to wrap my head around Jason's story, I struck up a conversation with Noah*, who was at the clinic with his new puppy. Also a veteran, Noah picked the breed because of their reputation as alarm barkers, and sleeps facing windows and doors, so that he can sleep more than an hour at a time.

Noah decided to get a puppy, because he thought it would be best knowing that when they walked, everyone would be watching the puppy, rather than the Marine.

A beautiful ranch home on top of a hill with a wrap-around porch and picture windows. To you and me, a perfect spot to sip coffee and watch the sunrise, or unwind with a bourbon brown ale and watch it set. To a retired Iraq veteran, a 360-degree view so as to defend against sneak attacks.

The last weekend in May is the unofficial start of summer and the official start of insanity for stir-crazy students and their teachers. The Monday that follows is Memorial Day. We are obliged to honor the memory and recognize our deep debt of gratitude to the military men and women who never returned home.

To have enlisted, served and survived can be an act of legacy, patriotism, purpose or valor. To return with soul intact and untouched

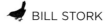
BILL STORK

is unthinkable. From WW II, through Vietnam and up to Afghanistan there are men and women who have returned with their lives, in no way shape or form, intact. While living day to day in security and freedom, the very least we can do is listen to their stories, internalize their struggles and be genuinely and thoughtfully thankful to our Veterans.

We would be well-served to meet their eyes and nod, shake a hand, or hug a soldier who has served our country, and as a consequence lives in fear of an "Extra Value Meal."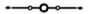

Names and minor details have been changed in this story to protect privacy.

Addendum: To hear one of the most heartbreaking songs ever written in homage to a veteran...

Fred Eaglesmith, "The Rocket." http://www.youtube.com/watch?v=DIfF8x55M0E

Black, White and Red

A dam and his mom Tracy were nearly out the door. He did an about-face, walked with purpose back into the room and offered me a handshake, full and firm. He thanked me, for a Kleenex.

Only a few hours before, Adam and Tracy had presented their 19-year-old cat named Red. He was profoundly dehydrated, and had lost his energy and half his body weight. The labwork made for a clear diagnosis. Telling Adam was painful. Red was in kidney failure. His prognosis was grave; his days were numbered. Adam listened intently as I described the disease process. Adam had never known life without Red. He rearranged the blankets that surrounded him, petted him vigorously, photographed and videoed. Finally, he kissed Red on the head, and left.

In a few months, Adam will begin his freshman year at Johnson Creek High School. He will take his place alongside the other academically gifted kids in honors math and science. A point of pride for any family; an achievement of monumental proportions for Adam and his family.

At 2-1/2 years of age his parents recognized that Adam struggled with communication and language. After a series of misunderstandings and misdiagnoses, Adam, thanks largely to his dad's tenacity, was diagnosed with Asperger's syndrome, a form of Autism. Adam sees things as black and white, right and wrong. Unfortunately, instead of leading to treatment, diagnosis only helped Adam and his family understand.

Adam has taught himself how to function in a world that is often nothing short of chaos, an amazing feat of strength and courage. Yet he is a boy who struggles with input, even from those who love and care for him the most. Red was always there. He always listened, always agreed and never talked back. The value of a friend like Red is beyond measure.

As he left the clinic, Adam thanked me for offering a Kleenex to dry his tears, as he said goodbye to his best friend. Well Adam, we thank you and Red, for helping to define the value of human-

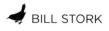 BILL STORK

animal interdependence, and for motivating us to do our very best for every animal at the other end of our stethoscope. Thank you for being a 14-year-old example of strength in the face of adversity.

You will never forget Red, and we will never forget you. ⟨⊙⟩

So Thankful

We are eternally grateful for all our clients, not the least of which is Jean Jensen.

In any given visit Jean will express that she is "so thankful" for anyone from her boss to the young woman who checked her groceries. This story and several more could be filled with a bullet-point list of all the things Jean Jensen is thankful for.

Though giving thanks is her favorite topic of conversation, she never fails to inflect. She will first bow her head slightly, and then turn right and left. "I'm telling you, Dr. Stork," she rocks forward on the bench. Palms inward and shoulder width, she punches the hard first consonants like a conductor, "I am so thankful." She raises her eyes, rolls back and crosses her hands over her chest, as she elaborates in detail what she is grateful for.

Well Jean, 'tis the season, and today we turn the tables and say we are "so thankful" for you.

In February 2011, Jean stopped by the Dane County Humane Society, "just to take a look." She held the door for a sobbing young mother and her daughter, there to surrender the family cat.

Sierra was nearly ten years old, with dental disease, a chronic skin condition and a future that was anything but hopeful. Her family had been double-punched in the bottom of the recession, struggling to provide for themselves, and unable to care for Sierra. Jean could have adopted any cat. Without hesitation, she took Sierra into her arms, and the family under her wing.

For Sierra, she has provided medical care and a wonderful home. For the family she scours rummage sales and second-hand shops for children's clothes and provisions. In the nearly two years since they met in the vestibule of the humane society, the family has found work and gotten back on their feet. On a day when they most needed a smile, Jean was there.

 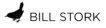 BILL STORK

Jean has worked as a Teller at US Bank on the Capitol Square in Madison. She engages the young people who come to her window. In turn, they share their achievements and challenges. Memorable to me was a young man who withdrew a sizeable sum of his summer's wages. His family had little to look forward to and he had worked, earned and saved enough to take his brother and sister to Great America before school started.

We know these things because she tells us, often without so much as raising her eyes from her knitting as she waits for our technicians to return Sierra from her procedure. She could just as well tell us whether she had whole wheat or sourdough toast for breakfast. Helping people is simply who she is.

Any day that Jean walks through your door is better than when she does not. There is no shortage of people helping and being kind. A fine commitment for any of us, on the eve of Thanksgiving, would be to borrow a page from the woman who is perpetually So Thankful.

Happy Thanksgiving from the staff of the Lake Mills Veterinary Clinic.

Olé, Silver Anniversary Edition

Some lessons should last a lifetime. You may recall that while still in school doing a midnight calf check, I was distracted by a friend and classmate. Only to be rescued by the very source of the distraction, after a Hereford cow unceremoniously tossed me against a wall. Every 25 years, an opportunity for a refresher comes along.

Monday, June 17, 2013, started like any other. Alarm sounds at 4:43 a.m., 3-year-old Australian Shepherd-Blue Heeler crawls next to me for a little head scratch, and feet on the floor. No need for a snooze alarm: a 48-year-old bladder takes care of that just fine.

As a clear manifestation of "nature and nurture." my chosen wake-up and rack out times are both predestined and calculated.

First, my grandpa was one generation physically removed from the family farm, and a millwright at the A.E. Staley Corporation in Decatur, Illinois. For those of you from south of the (Wisconsin) border, the birthplace of the Chicago Bears. He may have been the first to prove you can take the boy off the farm, but you can't take the farm out of the boy. He'd rise in time to go to the lake, catch a mess of crappie, filet and freeze 'em, and punch the clock at 8:00 a.m.

This trait would later save his life. Well before dawn on July 8, 1974, two rail cars full of propane gas collided and punched a hole in one. Being the closest house to the explosion, Grandpa's bedroom wall collapsed. Thankfully, Grandpa had taken his seat on the throne. A warm, mid-summer day, the window behind him was open. Before he could get to Ann Landers' solution for a marriage gone cold, he found himself sitting in the side yard, with the window frame at his feet.

Second, the specific time is thanks to one of my most favorite farm clients. Marilyn Claas farmed for the better part of 50 years with her husband and kids, the last few of which were solo, as her husband passed early of leukemia. "Stubborn" isn't so flattering; my dad calls that defining trait "German Persistence." Being a strong woman and wife, she vowed to keep working until the farm was

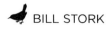 BILL STORK

paid for. Marilyn got to the barn early, so when cows had trouble, she would call by 5:00 a.m.

I consider myself generally a person of good nature, so long as I get two bowls of Corn Flakes, a glass of orange juice and a cup of coffee on the front end of whatever happens next. I tried 4:30, but was exhausted by the end of the day. If I lay around until 4:45, I find myself playing catch-up. After careful research, I concluded that Reveille at 4:43, and I am out the door and ready to roar.

Mrs. Claas has not milked a cow in nigh on to 20 years, but old habits don't die. When the phone doesn't ring, you have a built-in piece of unobstructed time to research cases, split firewood, fix the tractor or ride your bike.

On June 17, the phone did ring, just as I rinsed my cereal bowl. The first known destination for that mid-summer morning was to have been a herd health check, 40 minutes north and east. There was a moment of consternation when Butch Spiegelhoff called. His farm is just south of Columbus, 40 minutes to the north and west. Butch hasn't milked a cow in over 20 years either, but he has two herdsmen who do, and he had a cow struggling to deliver twins.

The 2011 Cummins Turbo Diesel has some pretty good snort if you've got a mobile veterinary hospital and need to get to a farm in a hurry. Not to mention, we don't really blend in with the Ford Escapes and Toyota Camrys. I make sure the little portable reminders by the side of the road don't flash at me when I'm just goin' for groceries, hoping to build a little cred so that when Officer Bob sees a white flash across his dash he knows there's blood spurtin'. On this day, time was at a premium, and unbeknownst to me as I flew past houses farms and fields, the morning would get more urgent, even before Butch's twin heifer calves were on the ground.

I made the hard left into Butch's drive a little hot, the ¾ ton truck fishtailing in the muddy drive like a late model on a dirt track. The breast pocket zipper on my coveralls was incontinent, so rather than risk a "Dr. Clark" and drop my cell phone in the stainless steel bucket full of disinfectant, I rested it on the flat spot on the dash board. Whatever came next would have to wait until Butch's cow had birthed.

Most cows that struggle to deliver twins do so as a result of presentation. Like brothers fighting over a toy truck, the calves compete for who gets the first birthday. The hard part is usually figuring out which feet belong to the head you're feeling. In this case, it was all about size. Both calves were big enough to wean.

The delivery went smoothly. Equipment was cleaned and back in the truck in short order. Butch's dad was a WWII Veteran and professional bike racer, so there are plenty of opportunities for distraction on the Spiegelhoff farm. Today we moved with purpose, so that the herdsman at the Griswold farm 50 minutes away would not have to wait for his herd check.

As I fell in behind the wheel and tore out the drive, I was pleased with progress. That euphoria would prove to be short-lived, as the little green message light was flashing on the phone.

The only known farm north of my current location was Matt Dams. Since it wasn't midnight, I knew he wouldn't call, so I drove southward and waited for the first piece of straight road to retrieve the messages, rather than risk hanging by my seatbelt in the middle of a plowed field.

The bad news: there were four of them. The good news: they were all from the same rather excitable farmer. In order to preserve anonymity we will only say the calls were from our most tenured technician. She and her brother milk 50 cows near Watertown. Both are quite capable, yet prone to panic when the wheels start to wobble.

Every herd has a personality. Here is a farm where one would be safer in full-on NHL issue goalie gear. This day was to be different. It was a heifer attempting to calve, in the open face building near the barn. She had yet to join the gang. Sheila, being cautious by nature, and deeply concerned about he who signs her paycheck, identified the expectant heifer as a pet.

As we approached she was lying in a deep pack of corn stalks, peacefully straining every few minutes. In the event she should stand, I suggested we put a halter on her head. If she decided to roam, we could anchor her. As I approached with the halter, she stretched and stood. She ambled slowly as we positioned the rope

 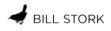 BILL STORK

behind her ears and over her nose. The calf was already out to the neck and shoulders. The delivery would be a cinch, but would require that I be behind her. Like two 5th graders ballroom dancing in gym class, she kept me squarely in her sights, and waltzed to a 3/4 rhythm only she could hear.

As I picked the post where I would tie her, I spoke gently and tugged at the rope. Somehow I figured she would follow along like a Standard Poodle just back from Westminster. Instead, she continued her amble with little regard for me or my halter. Not a surprise, as most cattle not halter-trained for the county fair don't exactly sit, stay, or heel. So, I braced my boots in the bedding and commenced pulling her to the wall.

In an instant, the game changed.

She turned like a rodeo bull. Her left eye turned to find a target, while I faced the business end and the dangling calf. She let go with both back feet. Thankfully I am blessed with the reflexes of a glacier, so I stood-stock still. Her hocks parted the wind like a whiffle ball bat, and whooshed past my ears.

By now, Sheila had tapped out. From over the gate she cackled like Edith at Archie, "Git outa they'a, she's gonna keel you!"

Getting out seemed appealing for the moment, but would by definition create a secondary dilemma: how to get back in the pen. After all, she still had a calf flailing from her vulva. Not to mention, I had folks waiting on me, and this was getting personal.

"Those who ignore the past, are doomed to repeat it."

Having established that any tension would escalate her, I clung loosely to the end of the rope and made subtle movements backing her up until I had enough slack to fish the rope around a sturdy post, which was tight to the tin skin of the barn.

Once accomplished, there would be one last round. The goal was to snub her nose tight to the wall, so Sheila could inject a half mL of sedative she had gotten from the truck to slow her down and level the playing field. If it were legal, and she weren't averse to needles, I might've recommended 5cc of Valium for Sheila.

Ms. Hyde pawed the bedding like a Brahman who had just thrown a cowboy 3.5 seconds into the ride. Stalks flew over her back, head low and cocked. The staff of Aesculapius embroidered on my chest was squarely in the middle of her 300-degree field of vision. I wrapped the rope once around my upturned palm for maximum power and easy exit, and squatted low. Like tackle tug-o-war at the Labor Day picnic, I heaved... and so did she: out of her stance like Clay Matthews on an all-out blitz.

She uppercut my ribs in sequential blows, just as I'd planned. With each thrust she gave me more slack to pull her closer, and in seconds, she was nose to nose with a 6x6.

Sheila injected her with the Xylazine. Within minutes the calf was born. That evening and to this day, "Ms. H." walks in the barn and milks as peacefully as a nun.

Sheila's threats of death by heifer were grossly exaggerated and thankfully inaccurate.

Four sore ribs, 800mg of Ibuprofen and we were back at it; an hour and a half late for the herd check, but no worse and maybe a bit wiser. ❧

 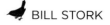

Old Dogs, New Tricks

It has been said for generations that "you can't teach an old dog new tricks." At the risk of outing husbands who don't help with the dishes, we beg to differ.

Countryside Jewelry has been a fixture in downtown Lake Mills for the better part of three decades, largely thanks to the owner and jeweler-in-residence, John Black. Coincident with the peak color of the majestic maple on the corner of Lake and Main in clear view from the picture window of the storefront, John is known to go missing each year, having traded his khakis and jeweler's loupe for hunting vest and shotgun. Twenty yards in front of him is 48 lbs of liver, white, and perpetual motion.

Hunting since the day she was weaned, if it's hatched and flies, it will be flushed, pointed and retrieved. A passionate and skilled hunter, John often hosts his college buddies for weekends afield. Long before they've taken the edge off Chase, you will find the party in front of the Packers game and a bowl of chips. At ten years of age there is absolutely no sign of her slowing down.

As indefatigable as Chase is in the field, it is not her only skill. She is equally enthusiastic in her ability to grow toenails, and her resistance to having them trimmed. We at the Lake Mills Veterinary Clinic take as our mission to deliver the most complete and compassionate care possible, and to do so in a manner that causes owner and pet as little stress as possible. We call it the behavioral approach, conceived and guided by our staff behaviorist, Mittsy Voiles.

Mittsy has developed a repertoire of techniques that have, over time, changed the nail trimming process from a cage match to a yoga session. Unique methods that have worked fabulously on scores of dogs; methods that Chase has systematically dismantled in a fraction of a second each. As a result, Chase's nail trims had come to involve 2-3 Certified Veterinary Technicians, one Certified Professional Dog Trainer, and one Doctor of Veterinary Medicine, who outweighs Chase by a factor of 5. And about 10 pounds of treats.

No one was in danger of being bitten. Chase simply had no intention of staying in one spot long enough to think about trimming a nail. The appointments were always entertaining; where and how her nails would be trimmed was anyone's guess. Once Chase wrapped herself around my neck, as if she was stuck in a tree, but the position was not to be duplicated.

And then we learned that Chase will negotiate, as long as the treats are good enough. Loaded with treats, Mittsy placed a blanket on the floor and sat down. Chase came over, and sat on the blanket. "Good girl," followed by a treat, and the game was on. Mittsy touched Chase's shoulder. Chase, intent on the treat bucket, sat calmly without moving away. Another treat! Mittsy lifted Chase's paw — no reaction, another treat! And thus they progressed. Chase pulled her paw away once, and Mittsy let go of it, but Chase got no treat for that round. Chase quickly realized that holding still for short moments earned a treat, and no one would hold her down.

Progressing from touch-treat to clip-treat was a cinch. We accomplished her nail trim in 5 minutes, with zero restraint and one staff member (although the others hung around like the gallery at the Masters — each successfully trimmed nail drew a gasp and a soft clap).

In this season of appreciating tradition, we are nonetheless happy to bid goodbye to our longstanding ritual of all-hands-on-deck for Chase's nail trim, and to welcome an opportunity to spend more time scratching her ears and catching up with John.

 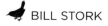

And Then There Was Light

L ake Mills Veterinary Clinic had been closed twice in 20 years. Thursday, December 20, was number three. We tried. All staff not 8 months pregnant or ravaged with flu reported for duty, on time. Not the least of whom was technician Kelly, who has recently returned from a year in Alabama, and warms her car for 15 minutes when the temperatures dip below 50 F.

Our first sign of things to come could have been when we had to get our snowplow driver out of bed; he had just assumed we would be closed like everyone else. The day began reasonably enough. A few inches of wet snow and a 10mph wind from the NW were nothing the local fleet of F-250s s couldn't clean in one sweep, with their window still rolled down.

By noon it got serious. Snowflakes the size of quarters were being driven horizontal. The flakes that landed in our parking lot must surely have left the sky over Lake Superior. With temperatures still hanging in the low 30s, you were either going to break the handle out of your shovel or lumbar vertebra 5.

When our head technician's mother called at 3 p.m. and said something to the effect of, "Tell Dr. Stork he's crazy and you girls get your butts home," the decision was made.

With traction and visibility at a premium, maximum speed on the 8-mile-drive home was 35mph.

The frozen load proved too much for the power lines. When I hit the button to open the garage, nothing happened. In the face of the blizzard, it seemed unthinkable we would have electricity before tomorrow. We budgeted remaining daylight to start a fire and located the mountain microwave (Dutch oven) to heat leftovers. Horses, goats, cats and dogs were fed and watered. Now to clear snow.

By the time I made the top of the driveway, the only sounds were the howl of the wind and the rhythmic tight growl of the little John Deere. The only light was the occasional yellow roller on the county plow truck and cold, steel-blue flashes of lightning across the night sky. The little house sat cold and dark at the bottom of the hill. As I surveyed my handiwork, warming my hands in the diesel exhaust, an ambulance broke the silence, moving as fast as they could safely travel. At the same time, the Christmas lights above our sun room flickered to life.

It is worthy of a pause. Thanks to someone, somewhere, 40 feet high in a driving snowstorm in a bucket truck, 2,500V of electricity in each hand, I'm able to write this little piece in a warm, well-lit house. Thanks to a crew of city, state and county workers and a fleet of plow trucks, that ambulance was able to get to a patient in need. As the sun comes up tomorrow, we will all be able to hit the road to work and school. Thanks to all who make that happen. ❧

 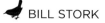 BILL STORK

Blood Red, Pasty White and Screaming the Blues

I have climbed some of the most spectacular high mountain passes in all the United States. Black Bear pass near Telluride, Stony Pass near Silverton and Liberty pass near Gunnison, to name a few. It can be said that none would have been possible, had I not first conquered a quarter mile field road with 400 ft of elevation gain near the southern terminus of Newville Road.

Equally true is that the view from 13,000 feet on the Continental Divide is no more spectacular than the blinding green and rolling fertile fields and forests surrounding the little shack at the top of Bauriedel's Hill.

I can't honestly say I leapt from my lawn chair and clapped for joy when the phone rang, but I knew there would be payoff beyond calf birth.

As the sun began to sink into the western haze early in the evening of our nation's 220th birthday, Butch called. He had a cow that was having trouble, "out back."

For those more confined to the concrete, there is a rule with regard to cows on pasture. You could plant one rosebush on one end of a hundred-acre pasture and put a cow on the other. When it came time to calve, she would seek the prickly bush, back into it, and commence labor.

My powder blue half-ton Chevy work truck growled and lurched up the rutted, winding dirt road. I pulled her into granny low and set the brake on the closest thing I could find to a flat spot, crossing my fingers the transmission would hold her there. Long since having grown over, there once was a 6x8 gateway through the white pines at the clinic, a testament as to the security of the parking brake I kept meaning to have fixed.

With no sign of Butch, and the grass armpit-high, I climbed onto the roof of my truck to find the one rose bush the cow was assuredly trying to calve into. A hundred yards in the distance, I saw my patient. Setting my bucket, rope, meds and calving tool next to the three-wire electric fence, I rolled underneath, situated my gear and hiked over to her.

True to form, there she lay — head uphill, with her birthing parts nestled into the base of a twelve-foot tall, multiflora rose bush. Gifted to Wisconsin Dairy farmers by the Department of Agriculture to be used as line fences 75 years ago, words to describe my counter proposal are not suited for family publications.

Thankful once again that my dad worked construction, and I was familiar by association with the use of levers and elevation, with a 3/4 inch rope halter, a nearby scrub oak and a modicum of youthful gumba, I was able to peewhistle her onto her side and pivot her downhill, rendering her free from the bush.

(Peewhistle being a construction term, usually a verb, meaning to change direction. In the most strict sense, this maneuver was actually a compound peewhistle. You move the piece, in the case a cow, from where it is to where you need it to be.)

When I rotated her out of the bush, she was then pointed downhill, disadvantageous for both birth and hemodynamics (blood flow). So, with one last tug on her tail and bull hunch to her hip, she was sideways on the hill.

With only two of the calf's feet showing and pointed down, I stripped to the waist, gloved up and lay on my stomach, reaching for a head or tail. I found neither. Eventually, I located an eye socket and a nostril, and was able to palm the calf's head like a bowling ball, sweeping it into alignment between the two front feet. Once in position, with the assistance of a pair of chains and a few pulls, a star was born.

As expected, mom showed no attempt at trying to rise. I reached for my bucket and used what was left of the evening's light to set a 14-gauge needle in her right jugular. Crisis averted.

Coveralls rolled to my waist, I stood shimmering with blood, sweat and fetal fluid, admiring my handiwork and God's creations. As the medicine ran slowly into her vein and the newborn calf scrambled

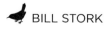 BILL STORK

to stand and nurse, the sky flashed with the Waterloo Volunteer Firemen's epic fireworks display.

Science has yet to determine whether ethnicity, diet, or body chemistry renders some more attractive to the mosquito than others. Let the record show that a properly marinated Eastern European flatlander, at sunset on top of a hill, is prime.

A gentle summer breeze from the west had apparently dispersed my essence. Before the medicine could drain into the cow's vein, every mosquito in Jefferson County was en route. Dancing, swatting and cussing at the onslaught, had I suffered a grand mal epileptic seizure it would have been more elegant. There are moments when it is every man and beast for themselves. That time was nigh.

Quickly making a sign of the cross in the cow's general direction, I slung the rope halter over my left shoulder and the calf jack over my right. For the first 25 meters, Usain Bolt would have been no match for me, as I high-stepped through the meadow, Lacrosse rubber overshoes for racing flats. As the truck came into view, a healthy half of Wisconsin's State Birds had made off into the night with my red blood cells. I became weak.

I heaved my tools under and dove through the wires of the fence. With bucket and box in the passenger side, I jumped under the steering wheel and reached to roll up the window, all the while screaming like a Jack Nicholson nightmare.

Lesson learned. From July 5, 1996 to present, from Easter to Thanksgiving the truck doesn't roll without at least a quart of 40% DEET under each seat, and in every door pocket. ❧

A Fair Legacy

Alongside rolling rural roads, you have surely noticed the square blue yard signs with white block letters that say "Fair."

Look closely, and you may see boys and girls sporting cut-off jeans and tank tops with knee-high brown rubber boots. 75-pound 7th graders hang onto one end of a shiny nylon show halter, with an 1,800 lb Angus steer on the other.

Smell closely, and you will see others with a long stick in their hand, a grimace on their face, and words unbecoming on their lips. These are the boys and girls showing pigs for the Meat Animal Project, attempting to impose their will on a 280 lb omnivore the Romans once used to plow rocky virgin soil.

By the time you are reading this, they will be penned or tied, shaved, scrubbed and on display in the barns on the north end of the Jefferson County Fairgrounds. Above them will be signs and sayings for their respective 4-H groups, and under them will be two feet of clean yellow straw or shavings. Behind them will be a sleep-walking kid waiting to escort the animal's next "movement" out of sight and smell, so that when mom and dad walk through with tired toddlers high on their shoulders there are more "awws, and "can we pet them?" than "P.U" through pinched nostrils.

Whether you are drawn to the fair for the Badger State Truck Pull, the Little Big Town concert, or fried Twinkies on a stick, budget a bit of time to absorb what a rural county fair is all about. Walk through the dairy, beef, swine, goat, poultry, rabbit and craft barns. I promise you will be in awe of some of the photographs on display. In my case, they were taken by friends I had known by way of their vomiting cat, and I had no clue they had ever picked up a camera.

Pause to appreciate a barn wood table crafted by a young man out of scraps of siding and fence posts from his grandparents' farm. Notice the detail of the dioramas created by kids, of the farms they grow up on, bale hay for, or visit. Look for a stunning cherry wood mandolin, every piece but the strings and frets made by a handy-

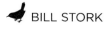 BILL STORK

man farm hand from just across the river, of wood salvaged from a Saturday night bonfire social.

There was a time when the county fair was the highlight of the year. Summer was brief, all about surviving winter, and planting, picking, mowing, baling, cutting, splitting, stacking and fixing. The fair was five days of rest, socializing, and maybe showing off a bit.

A few generations on, there are considerably fewer folks with calluses and cow manure. That said, those hogs, steers and heifers don't just stand and lead by way of their good nature and the desire to please. It all begins when the snow still flies. The animals at show have been weighed, fed and recorded for months. As Fair time nears, kids court local business and service providers, shaking hands, taking pictures, and inviting interested buyers to see their animals on the farm.

All are hopeful that when their pig stands at the meat animal sale, and the Stade boys precede their machine-gun auction banter with, "Now there's a fine looking young lady, mighty proud of her hog," the bids come fast and furious. If all goes well, they'll cover their costs, plus a few weeks of college tuition.

Many kids who show learned from their parents, who in turn were inspired, motivated and instructed — if not prodded — by a somewhat maniacal FFA instructor named Lyle Wallace. Nearly every day of his summer was giving to kids. He would load his blue Ford station wagon and hurtle through the county roads. No doubt, at times caring more than they did, he ensured that every kid had blood samples, health papers and bidders for their animals. Without fail, there was a 50-cent ice cream cone from McDonald's at the end of the day.

Lyle Wallace did not invent agriculture, accountability or citizenship, but he represented them well. He and his wife were tragically killed in a car accident in 1997. Lyle and Becky left behind three exemplary children and a gymnasium full of students who have gone on to farms and families from Lake Mills to Rosendale and beyond. His kind of caring lives on to this day on the sidelines and practice fields of the Lake Mills varsity boys' soccer team.

"To live on in the hearts of those you leave behind, is to not die." I can think of no better time than — at an event he worked so hard for — to reflect and recall a man who for his students and family, gave it all. ◈

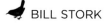 BILL STORK

Under Pressure. Or Not.

On May 15, 1992, I graduated from the University of Illinois – College of Veterinary Medicine. Seeking dairy cows, hills and freedom from Bears fans, I migrated across the Cheddar Curtain to take a job at the Lake Mills Veterinary Clinic. Immediately I found myself navigating my way medically and geographically, all while adjusting to a new dialect. I learned that when one is thirsty, you search for the nearest "bubbler." When your legs are tired, you sit on your "hinder."

Dr. Bruce Brodie taught us how to replace the uterus in a cow who had recently calved. Little did I know we would be asked to attend fresh cows who had "tossed their calf beds," or "cast their withers." So, when I learned that all pigs shown at the Jefferson County Fair were required to test negative for a disease called pseudorabies, my volunteering hand went up like a 5th grader with the answer. Well into his sixties, Dr. Anderson was school-girl-giddy at the chance to delegate the job to the rookie.

For the Meat Animal Project, young boys and girls seeking ribbons and a chunk of college money at the Jefferson County Fair house their pigs on grandparents' and friends' farms. They use anything from a re-purposed milking parlor, to a dilapidated lean-to, and a knee-deep bog.

It has been said, "Never teach a pig to sing, it wastes your time, and annoys the pig." Rest assured, they are even less thrilled at the notion of having blood drawn from their jugular vein. With all due respect to nurses charged with the responsibility of drawing blood from patients of all sizes, ages and attitudes, imagine, if you will, the pig. Weighing 250 lbs or more, pigs have an extremely low center of gravity, all-wheel drive and not a vein showing anywhere on their body. They are exquisitely designed to withstand attack from any pack of predators. A greenhorn vet, his sidekick FFA instructor with a funny mustache, and a station wagon full of students would seem not to have a chance.

To draw a blood sample from a pig, the pig must first stand still, which is not in their nature. A pig's version of human contact is taking small nibbles of your boots. Even when they have been hand raised, and taught to drive and stand on command, you're going to need some equipment, which can range from baler twine to a 4', retractable implement.

After much trial and experience, I can speak with authority: the tool of choice is an 8" snare, consisting of a 1/4" cable attached to a T-handle that runs through the long axis of a 3/8" L shaped pipe, then anchors to the short side to form a loop. You can buy them at Nasco for $30 or so, but the high-performance custom model from a jack of every trade named Dale, at the University of Illinois Swine Research Center works best. They can be purchased for a 6 pack of Miller Light.

The morning arrived. Lyle Wallace creaked into the parking lot just before 7:00, his Ford wagon shimmying with FFA kids hopped up on Mountain Dew, bumper nearly dragging. With half a smile and a swagger, I hung my arm out the window, cranked the morning program, and followed to the first farm.

Whatever Mr. Wallace lacked in boots-on-the-ground experience, he doubled in energy and enthusiasm. An educator to the core, all the world was his classroom. In a flash he took the snare from my hand and hurdled the first gate, hell-bent on demonstrating proper technique to his students.

One approach would have been for me to subtly suggest that, while curiosity may kill a cat, it is the very trait that would render a pig snared. But feeling the need to build a little cred, and oblivious to the travails that would soon befall me, I chose silence.

The goal is to slip the snare over the snout, behind their clipped canines. In doing so, they will immediately throw it into "4-low." That's when the catcher is engaged in a tug-o-war, and the phlebotomist slides in for the sample. Eventually Lyle would outlast our first patient, but not until he and the pig had lapped the pen a half dozen times, trashed his Levi's and bloodied his lip.

Vets from James Herriot to Kuffel had used a 6" harpoon and a 12cc syringe. Once snared, they would kneel before the pig and pull the sample from the cranial vena cava, centimeters from the heart.

 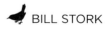 BILL STORK

A card-carrying graduate of the Dave Bane School of Porcine Phlebotomy, I chose a 1-1/2 inch needle, and a 7cc Vacutainer tube — identical to the rig used by nurses in hospitals. Once in the vein, you slide the rubber stopper over the opposite end of the needle, and the pressure created by the vacuum fills the tube with blood.

Choosing not to show my cards, I had been part of the core research establishing prevalence of the very disease from which we were saving the Jefferson County Fair. As students we would take several day trips deep into central and southern Illinois, often bleeding 600-1,200 pigs in a day.

A handful of students and two farmers leaned on the fence and spat. One Ag instructor grunted and panted on the handle, while the pig effortlessly tossed his head on the business end of the snare. I approached with all the confidence of someone who had conservatively bled 2,000 pigs.

Rotating my John Deere cap, I strode to the pig's right side. Kneeling, I gently placed my left fingertips in her thoracic inlet and slipped the needle squarely into her jugular vein, expecting a 20-gauge gusher.

Nothing happened.

I made subtle adjustments to free the tip of the needle from the wall of the vein. Like a 250 lb turnip, not a drop.

The most bloodshed was from Mr. Wallace's lip, as he had chased our first pig under the edge of a corrugated steel roof. Either Wisconsin pigs have dramatically different plumbing than their cousins to the south, or I was experiencing an equipment failure of epic proportions, before a live audience. Alas, no combination of needles or tubes in my pocket would render a red blood cell.

Mr. Wallace meanwhile, kept his good nature. As sweat sprang from his trembling forearms and his head grew progressively redder, he maintained his tug-of-war with the six month old Berkshire barrow.

Feeling like Geraldo looking for Hoffa, and fresh out of excuses or explanation, I squared my shoulders and resorted to the truth.

"I've bled a lot of pigs, and this has never happened," I explained. "Be back tomorrow," I promised.

Wondering if crow really tastes like chicken, I made the long slow drive back to the clinic. The radio was silent. As I related the experience to my boss, he asked to see the tubes I had used.

At a glance, he nodded. "You know, after you use those tubes the first time, you can clean 'em up, put on a new label and fill them again."

It has been said that copper wire was invented by two Scots, fighting over a penny.

Vacutainers cost about a nickel apiece. I had no way of knowing that Dr. Anderson had been cleaning and re-using them; rendering what was once a vacuum container, simply a glass tube.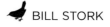

BILL STORK

Alice's Restaurant

The day-to-day of a country vet consists in no small part of driving in circles. There will be occasions of flash frustration and teeth gnashing, but it is for the better. Delivering mail it is not; some things you just can't schedule.

The day started at 6:00 a.m., writing health papers for county fair pigs in 'Crick. This was followed by treating an "under the weather" cow and a sore foot near Deerfield by 8:00. En route to herd check at Haack's by 9:00, and the phone vibrates to indicate a message has been left sometime during the last 30 minutes. Were it not 75 degrees and sunny, and my window not been rolled down as I headed west on Dane County BB; if Dallas Wayne had not played Steve Earl's Copperhead Road, I may have heard it ring.

I listen to the message. Gentleman Glenn has a heifer calving, and she's having trouble.

Mr. Rummler has 18 Angus pets with names they respond to, and they come for grain in the same wooden stanchions where he milked cows as a boy. In 75 years he has had one address, minus a tour of duty in Korea. There he served as an optics specialist in the Army. Glenn is as much a philosopher as a farmer and I get a subtle electric tingle under my collar at the notion the man should raise a glove off the wheel of his David Brown tractor when he sees me drive past to another farm.

This day I was feeling no less honored, yet not quite so charmed. From the roof of a 60-foot silo, I could have seen Glenn's farm, from where I had been just 90 minutes ago, on a day when I didn't exactly have the time to spare.

Backtracking to the Rummler Farm, I pass the first farm house I rented when I moved from the flatlands to America's Dairyland. Turn left and you will cross the bridge over I-94 where Steve's Car and Truck Service extracted a Kennworth sleeper cab wedged like a splittin' maul in a piece of oak.

To the west will be a field where Jim Erb was fall-plowing 20 years ago. By the time I had waved, driven the mile home and was through the first shower, there would be a message on the clinic phone. He couldn't wait to hear why I was driving around Jefferson County in my underwear.

Another quarter mile will bring you to Ranch Road. Turn right, and you are at the Rummler farm. Turn left and the road quickly dead-ends into the Johnson Creek Landfill.

Caterpillar D12 bulldozers like Tonka toys unroll black tarps the size of football fields. Fleets of green Waste Management trucks have collected, compacted and delivered hundreds of tons of refuse per day for over two decades.

Life is built around occasions that mark the passage of time. Births, baptisms, graduations and marriages all beg for us to pause and reflect. The capping of a landfill is no less momentous.

Woody Guthrie wrote the back-handed anthem to America, "This Land is Your Land." His son Arlo wrote "Alice's Restaurant." At an average of 18 minutes long, he is famous for musing, "If you are ever to write a song, make sure you are willing to perform it, every day, for the rest of your life."

For those not familiar, on a fateful Thanksgiving Day he visits his friend Alice. Alice lives in the bell tower of a church. Since they have removed the pews, there is plenty of room for garbage where they used to be. Thinking it the neighborly thing to do, they load a half a ton of garbage in a red VW Microbus, and head for the city dump. Where they encounter a sign that specifically states, dump closed on Thanksgiving. Having never heard of a dump closed on Thanksgiving, they strike out in search of somewhere else to put the garbage. So, off the side of a side road, at the bottom of a 15 foot cliff, they find another pile of garbage. Rather than bring that pile up, they throw theirs down and return to the church for a Thanksgiving dinner that could not be beat.

All was right with the world until the next morning when officer Obey called. There had been an envelope at the bottom of the pile of garbage with his name on it.

Well, Arlo, I know exactly how you must have felt.

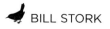 BILL STORK

You see, somewhere near the bottom of 25 years of garbage at the Johnson Creek landfill is a sale flyer from Bart's water ski supply. Postmarked late 1992, addressed to me, or resident. In Alice's Restaurant, which is not the name of the restaurant, but the name of his friend and the song, Arlo was arrested, interrogated and accused of dodging the draft. My crime was far less heinous, and the punishment would reflect. It did however, in the face of my best effort and intentions set me back 80 blue collar dollars, and thirty minutes of sanity.

In the fall of 1992 there was no single-stream recycling, curbside pickup or robotic garbage trucks in Farmington Township. The public landfill was open 8-noon, on even-numbered Saturdays. There was also far less cyber-commuting and flex-time at work for our clients. Often, Saturdays were the only time they could bring their pets in. For the vets and techs at the Lake Mills Veterinary Clinic, it was all hands on deck from the time you walked through the door. My garbage was of little concern to the cocker spaniel shaking her head and scooting on her backside.

The situation was critical. I had missed the last two dump days and was nearing Arlo's proportions. Loaded with a month and a half of our garbage, and the neighbor's as well. A retired painter and polka dancer, not in the least bit opposed to a midday Old Fashioned; six weeks of his recycling amounted to a bag or two of empty brandy bottles alone.

Critical Saturday arrived. We stacked the deck as best we could. Technician Sheila and I had provided the best service possible and stayed light on our feet. Still, it would be close.

I swerved out of the parking lot at 11:48 a.m., knowing the drive well and seldom making it in less than 15 minutes. With the urgency of a ruptured milk vein, I slid into the landfill at 12:04 p.m. Not a soul in sight. Where the dumpster had sat was an empty slot between two berms. The west for garbage; the east for recycling. New to the area, looking to do the right thing and not in the least looking forward to returning with all that rubbish, I contemplated. The fence was not too tall to heave the bags over and risk them bursting, and I could slip through the chained gate.

Taking into account contents and balance of the bags, and using meteorology to calculate the expected prevailing winds, I positioned them so as to require the least possible effort to nudge them in, when the dumpster returned. All while, taking minimal risk they would fall in and cause more work.

Unilateral as it may have been, pleased with my solution, I returned home for a Cheese Toasty (grilled cheese sandwich) that couldn't be beat, and a seven minute nap.

Six weeks later with the incident all but forgotten, I received a letter. A certified letter. Not from Officer Obey, but Farmington Town Clerk Bernice Sukow. An envelope with my name on it had been found in a bag, illegally dumped at the landfill.

I contemplated telling her the truth, that I had been missing such an envelope, and thanking her for locating it. I just could not bring myself.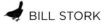

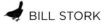 BILL STORK

Sneezing Cow

Happy New Year, and welcome to 2014.

At some point back in October this rank-amateur piece of small-town, pop psychological, feel-good rambling commemorated its third year. By my way of thinking, it is overdue (like the registration sticker on my license plate), to offer up some heartfelt gratitude.

First, to my editor, Mittsy Voiles, without whom any fifth grade English teacher would scratch this thing with enough red ink to float a 16-foot jon boat. I am at least as grateful to readers like, but not limited to, Don and Mary Grant, who will occasionally comment. The notion that we may have rendered a chuckle, a tear or someone may have seen beauty in life, is the ultimate reward. Fortunate, as we have yet to earn our first nickel.

Finally, and foremost, I am eternally grateful — in chronological order — to John-Boy Walton and Michael Perry. Thursday nights in the 70's I would push back from the table, clear dishes for Mom and help Dad in the garage, double-time, to ensure I was in front of CBS by 7:00. Minutes after Richard Thomas had scratched the morals of the week onto the parchment with his fountain pen 'neath the light of a single candle, I would scamper upstairs to my own diary.

In the 35 years to follow, I found myself in a perpetual cycle of going to school, graduating, getting educated, and meeting the most amazing people imaginable. The notion of writing was little more than a passing thought. Four years ago I read the book I always intended to write: a near biblical account of rural humanity called *Population 485*. This column and the blog from which it is extracted was born.

For anyone mildly entertained by our little column, but not familiar with Michael Perry, I ask that you put this paper down. Use the ten minutes to read Mike's Sunday column in the *Wisconsin State Journal* called "Roughneck Grace." Next to your "throne" keep a copy of "Off Main Street" or "Truck." If you don't find yourself belly laughing and crying, I'll buy the books back.

Mike was raised on a dairy farm in Northern Wisconsin; he and his family still reside near Eau Claire. He makes his living touching people. Writing, telling stories, and singing in his band "The Long Beds," Mike is as poetic as profound, setting forth such enduring wisdom as:

"Never stand behind a sneezing cow."

For anyone who has ever so much as set boot on a dairy farm, this seems pretty intuitive. By way of observation, and confirmed by Rick Schultz, Jake Untz and Ryan Haack — dairymen with collectively a century of experience — cows are not known to telegraph. Careful scientific research, in the sense that I asked every farmer I talked to last Thursday, concludes that the likelihood of being pasted is in direct proportion to the size of your herd and time spent in the barn. There are a few confounding variables, such as condition of your free stalls, the cow's diet, and your personal foot speed.

The Holstein (or to preempt an uprising from Carrie and Claire), the Dairy Cow has been referred to as "The Foster Mother of the Human Race." Centuries of conscientious breeding has rendered an animal that can produce in excess of 15 gallons of milk per day. She eats more than 100 pounds of feed and drinks 50 gallons of water.

Well, what goes in, must come out.

Cows live protected from moisture and draft on sand free-stalls, designed to encourage them to lay, and are groomed at each milking. In order to keep them clean, the bed is elevated by at least 8 inches. In pursuit of ultimate cow comfort, we have managed to position her "outlet." depending upon age, breed and facilities and adjusted for the stature of the farmer... about ear-hole high.

Sparing the details of bovine respiratory physiology, sneezing is a nearly spontaneous act. A forceful exhale against a closed glottis can propel 12 pounds of "effluent" at a velocity and viscosity sufficient to penetrate every pore. In the absence of a seasonally appropriate Green Bay Packers or drug company freebie hat, it will saturate you to the scalp. To exist within a 120-degree radius and 6 feet is to be in range. If you look down and find your bootlace

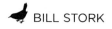 BILL STORK

untied... step away before retying it. You can take my word, or ask Charlie Untz.

On Monday, December 23rd, I spent two hours behind no fewer than 1,000 cows, each and every one eligible to sneeze without warning or provocation. The Gods and Odds of bovine respiration and digestion were kind on that day. I was spared a direct hit, which is not to be mistaken for "show room clean." I wished Rick and Kevin a Merry Christmas, scrubbed my boots and strode through the blowing snow to my truck.

I had four farm calls to go, it was three days before Christmas, and Boom-truck, Dusty and Go-Go (aka "big butt"), were short on horse feed. Farm and Barn was exactly en route. The dictum of the gentleman farmer and old school veterinarian requires you never appear in public with enough evidence of excrement to be detected by CSI; a noble notion, which I work hard to uphold. On this day, in the driving snow, disrobing in the slop of the parking lot was going to cost more time than I had. Not to mention, I was picking horse feed from a farm store, not hand lotion from *Bath and Body Works*.

What I failed to consider is, it was three days before Christmas, and school was out. The Salvation Army bell ringer was dressed in full-on Santa regalia and moms were pouring through the front door, hand in hand with daughters.

Unfazed, moving with purpose and thinking hard, I helped an elderly farmer throw a dozen bags of barn lime in his truck, and pilfered his four wheel flat-bed cart. Sparing the public exposure at the front door, like Eddie Lacy waiting for his blockers, I paused as the electric OUT door sprung open.

Wishing Christmas greetings to one and all, I shot past the only closed cash register and across the head lanes, straight for the power tools, certain I would find equally soiled brethren. Instead, there was a traffic-jam of moms and daughters. In solidarity with some really lucky fathers, I had to smile as they loaded the DeWalt 20-volt lithium ion drill and impact wrench package. Nevertheless, I was forced to re-route.

Lowering my head like an ostrich, I bolted past the paint section to the safety of tires and batteries. The waters parted, and I could see clear to the farm feed and mineral blocks. Certain they couldn't be serious about the 300 lb weight limit, I threw on 7 bags of "Veterinarian Approved Safe Choice," and reversed my path.

The register had extra room for wide loads, and was Command Central for a bespectacled lady named Dianne, with a permanent smile. Only two guys paying cash for a pocket full of gate pins and a battery for their 4-wheeler stood between me and the parking lot.

I threw three weeks' worth of equine vittles in the back seat and headed West on County 19, pleased with myself and convinced I had left "not a trace." Meanwhile, a four foot buffer zone around a slowly settling vapor trail, from farm supplies through auto parts, would suggest the contrary. ➣

 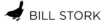

FDNY*

Whether you are Jed Hirschi herding 400 head of beef cattle across 90,000 acres of Wyoming on a Quarter Horse named Torque, or Ellen Messmer walking 18 Holstein dairy cows into a stanchion barn with a leather boot lace, moving cattle is a form of performance art. With a half step left, and a hand waved low, we steer the 1,200 lb ruminants, convincing them that's where they were planning to go anyhow. Calm as a yoga session in a mountain town.

Every cowboy and dairyman (and woman) has their own pet phrases and endearing style. Clem "the friendly monster" calls 'em "Camels." Mr. Behm refers to his "Kids." Many do it well, but none with more color than Brian Zabel.

For Brian, every milking was an Oscar-worthy performance in the category of "Spoken Word." Like a turn of the century European cattle drover meets Howlin' Wolf, he would start low and moan, politely suggesting it was time to get up and be milked. He'd nudge them up from their 4-foot sand stalls like Billy Mays pitching the Cham-Wow: "C'mon now ladies, it's time to go to work!"

Singly and in groups of three, they filed into the cow alley, Brian and herd swaying in unison. They ambled and chewed while he commentated. Like Pavarotti doing play-by-play, "It's cold out here, and warm in there" he projected from his diaphragm. Holding on to the "cold" and "warm" for a full four beats, he'd turn the words down, then up.

In a barnyard baritone that could rattle a foot of snow off a tin roof, "There's some country music on the radio and a nice lady with soft hands. She'll clean you up and milk you out," as if they understood every hard Germanic consonant.

"I got some silage, second crop and a little high-moisture corn. I'll throw it in the mixer and have breakfast ready when y'all get done," he bargained. "How's that sound?" searching for approval. About then, one would turn his way to lick her flank and swish. "Alright now ma'am! You've got a deal."

Brian walked with purpose, shoulders forward for momentum, pigeon-toed, elbows tight and arms swingin'. Like a cowboy's hat, you knew it was Brian a hundred yards away in the fog. His shoulder dropped a tick with the fall of his left foot; more of a hitch than a limp. It could have been courtesy of a cow last week or a full-back in high school. It was not about to break his stride and had never concerned him enough to take an Advil, let alone an X-ray.

Ask any country vet. They'll tell you the pager never sounds when you are sitting in your coveralls and boots, sipping coffee with your truck warmed up thinking, "Man, I've got a powerful hankering to go pull a calf right about now." It'll be about the time you step out of the shower, when the charcoal is about ready for the rib-eyes, ten minutes after you're snoring and drooling, or when your girl sits down and pulls back her hair to expose that spot on the back of her neck that's been aching all day.

In twenty two years we've gone from touchtone phones and an answering machine, through the age of the pager and now we have hand held computers with caller ID and GPS. Regardless, the term "grace" does not always describe the first reaction to an emergency farm call. There can be thoughts not consistent with the Veterinarian's Oath, words not suitable for the dinner table and on rare occasions, projectiles.

We remind ourselves the farmer didn't call because he had a good joke to tell, and he's been at it longer than you have. If the "911" came from Brian Zabel, you were particularly obliged to cut short the pity party, saddle up and get to work. Brian's "911" was always in form; a heartfelt acknowledgement of the intrusion, sandwiched between apologies.

"Good evening Dr. Stork! So sorry to interrupt the time with your lovely lady, Paige and Calvin, but we need some assistance with a brand new momma," he would boom with the enthusiasm of a Disney shuttle bus driver.

"I'm awfully sorry but I've tried everything and I'm gonna need an expert," like he hadn't pulled a thousand calves himself. From a man who is soaked through his insulated Carhartts, frozen to the bone and exhausted.

 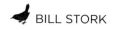 BILL STORK

In the time the frost clears the windshield, you find Del McCoury playing that high and lonesome sound on the radio. As fog clears the brain, you assemble your differential diagnoses, medicine and instruments. In the passing fields, corn stubble forms moon shadows on the January snow pack.

I can't imagine a Nobel Peace Prize sitting on the mantle would square my shoulders and clench my fist more than the experience of delivering a live heifer calf with Brian. Me, lying face down and armpit deep, searching for purchase and an extra pound of torque in order to bring up the southbound head of a northbound calf. Brian, wedged between a barn post and the cow's flank, straining like an Olympic power lifter to keep her from rolling on her side, and my right ear out of the manure and fetal fluid.

With the definition of insanity ("doing the same thing, expecting a different result") fully in play, we were one move away from a regroup, when the second knuckle of my left middle finger found the calf's right ear. With the last scrap of strength between the three of us, Brian rocked, the cow rolled and I heaved with a primal grunt. Tail-winded by some multi-denominational assistance, begged for from the Catholic on the ground and the Lutheran on the shoulder, the unborn calf, who would come to be known as "Wrong Way." was headed for daylight.

In short order we were shoulder to shoulder, each with a heifer's hock, draining the fluid from her lungs.

Brian was a hired man on a family farm. He was in the parlor by 3:30 in the morning, head down and hood up against the prevailing northwest wind. In his drafty rental house, his PJs were a clean pair of insulated Carhartts in order to save money and fuel. I did my dead level best to never arrive between noon and 2:00, as in the absence of unions and government mandates the farm hand split-shift is an hour for a sandwich and siesta.

Brian and the nice lady with the soft hands in the warm parlor had deep seated philosophical differences. She was an honorable John Deere woman, and he was an International Harvester man. After years of working cattle together, they were able to find middle ground. One fine spring day at the start line of the garden tractor pulling track at Utica Fest, they became husband and wife.

Both were offered jobs on a progressive organic farm in Grant County. My next encounter with Brian would be a decade later.

If I ever develop a seizure disorder, I know why. Parked in the far corner of the Kwik Trip parking lot, windows down for cross breeze, radio on low for an alarm, and just at the 4:30 point of a seven-minute nap, I felt a shoulder clasp and a resounding "DOCTOR STORK! Long time, no see."

In recent news, hundreds of New York City police officers and fire-fighters have been accused of fraud, claiming mental trauma sustained on September 11, leaving them unable to work, or so much as leave their homes. Coached by physicians and lawyers, these people were granted permanent disability and paid millions of tax-payer dollars, only to be found surfing, deep sea fishing and coaching martial arts.

People like Brian Zabel work to honor their industry, earn their credentials and contribute. They are not in pursuit of praise, promotion or a Christmas bonus; it's what they expect of themselves.

These people, on the other hand, expect less, much less. Their abhorrent actions only serve to magnify the sacrifice of the victims and bravery of the men and women of ...FDNY.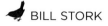

BILL STORK

The Great Alaskan Coffee Heist

Not much further than an Aaron Rodgers touchdown pass south of the intersection of Hwy BB and 73 is the Red Hip-Roof Dairy Barn of Wisconsin postcards, nestled under a knoll and protected from the west wind by a machine shed.

From the concrete pad next to the well head you take two steps down and 75 years back in time. Spare belts, rope halters and fencing supplies hang neatly. Straight on, a two-foot kitchen stand holds calf supplies, aspirin and a clear plastic tub of Tootsie Rolls or cashews. The south wall of the milk house, cleaner than Rachel Ray's kitchen, is decorated with framed awards for quality milk production.

For the past half-century and sadly for only a few months into 2013, 26 of the luckiest cows in the land have been tended by the hands of Larry and Betty Dahl. The first time I set my Lacrosse rubber overshoe on their farm and every visit since, I have been thoroughly humbled, charmed and enlightened. On the days when there is time beyond treating the cows, one usually gets back in the pickup with a belly laugh and a head shake.

Humbled, as anyone should be while standing on ground where Norwegian immigrants once stood. Rolling, rocky and wooded, they declared it a fine place to farm. A hundred and a half years later, there stand two homes, a dairy barn, and calf sheds; machine sheds full of tractors, wagons and spreaders; and a garage for farm trucks and the white Lincoln Continental Town Car for when you have to go to town.

Charmed, on my first visit watching Betty carry a Surge bucket back to the transfer. It was June and her sweat-soaked, V-neck t-shirt featured her bulging biceps and deltoids. I smiled to appreciate the results of hard life on the farm. And, I learned, a life membership to Princeton Club — all the better to keep a stranglehold on her title as National Arm Wrestling Champion.

Enlightened, on topics ranging from successfully maintaining a marriage and waking your mate in a manner that says, "I Love

You" without speaking the words. And medicine: "Vodka, with a hint of lemon for prevention; brandy, just a little warm, with honey, when you feel something comin' on."

For a guy who worked hard to never leave the farm, Larry seems to know a lot about what's going on in the world, and has a lot of friends in faraway places. Among the more memorable is his friend Dave, who lives in Alaska. Since winters aren't enough of a challenge in Anchorage, Dave has a place up Nort'.

Here in Wisconsin you don't get braggin' rights until you are north of Wausau. The alphas roam the woods of Eagle River and the UP. Dave, on the other hand, has an Alaskan cabin only accessible by snowmobile, 75 miles up a frozen river.

One can speculate that contractors, plumbers and electricians are scant in Dave's neighborhood, so he probably built the place himself. We can also assume it is void of luxuries such as indoor plumbing. Curbside garbage and recycling? Not likely.

On this trip, Dave had burned through supplies, firewood, and his yearning for solitude. Having had a highly successful 10 days of trapping and hunting, he packed for a morning departure. Nighttime temperatures had dropped to double digits below zero, and the first number was not 1.

The fetal position in his sleeping bag, wearing polypro, stocking hat and smart wool socks, was survivable. In the cabin one could easily see their breath, if there was light.

At just the time, too early to get up when the fire in the stove had dwindled a faint glow, nature called. The outhouse, ten yards out the door, was not an option. Legend has it that Paul Bunyan could flick a light switch and be in bed asleep before it got dark. Babe's master had nothin' on Dave.

With little time to negotiate, a decision was made to sacrifice the remnants of Folgers Breakfast Blend. The 2 lb can became a receptacle, and he was back in his cocoon.

Sleep would be elusive and light is brief in the Alaskan winter. Eventually Dave would gather his gear, and head for civilization.

 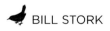 BILL STORK

Having successfully traversed the river, he loaded his snowmobile, packed his truck, and headed home. In need of food, fuel and a good stretch, he made a stop.

As America's "Last Frontier." there's not a Kwik Trip and McDonalds every eight miles. His yearn for solitude had been satiated, replaced by the pull of a hot meal and a friendly face. So when Dave saw the dim glow advertising fried chicken and mashed potatoes for $5.99, he pulled into the gravel lot, between mountains of plowed snow. In exchange for $8.00 and a detailed wildlife report including moose and bear sightings and tracks, Dave got a full belly and a smile.

The smile wouldn't last long. In America's Last Frontier we usually don't think in terms of security, but when Dave returned, his truck had been broken into.

As he circled his rig to check his load he saw the light of the diner shining through the corner of his camper shell. He turned the latches and shone his headlamp into the bed of the truck. Evidently in Alaska, though rare, roadside thieves are utilitarian, principled and wear size 11 shoes. Untouched were campstoves, guns and pelts hard-earned on trapping lines.

Missing were leftover steel-cut oats, 1/3 of a jar of peanut butter, his sleeping bag and snow boots. Violation and anger were but a flash as Dave recognized the missing supplies were tools of survival.

Dave's sense of bewilderment gave way to a commanding guttural belly laugh, as he realized that also missing was a "two-pound" can of Folgers Breakfast Blend. ◈

Mary Christmas

She thumped her tail twice, in response to the click of the catch as the storm door settled shut behind us. Through the screen a hundred-year-old maple filtered the late morning sun. I knelt and stroked her head, searching for what was left of muscle, and words that might comfort. Maybe to make it easier on Dave and me, she did not so much as flinch when I injected the sedative.

In minutes her eyes drifted shut. His left hand cradled her head while his right stroked her muzzle, as he lay nose to nose on the sweaty concrete. I slipped the 20-gauge needle into her vein and pushed. As I watched her chest over the top of my glasses, she took one last breath and relaxed.

For 14 years she made sure the cattle were on the right side of the fences and strangers never got out of their cars. Today, she retired.

As we stood, I opened my eyes wide, and exhaled, shook his callused hand and clasped the shoulder of the third generation dairy farmer. We rounded the garage together and I started for my truck. As I stowed my gear, Dave crossed the drive, collapsed on the porch and dropped his head to his upturned palms. I grabbed the steering wheel and had one foot in the truck, but the empty space next to him on the wooden step felt like a friend in need. I walked back, sat and stared at the alfalfa until his chest stopped heaving, and he came up for air.

There are herd dogs, hunting dogs, lap dogs and pets. For many, they are truly man's best friend. For a few, they are God-sent saviors.

It was early winter 1988. The barn radio sat between the rafters, frozen on "Janesville and Southern Wisconsin's home for country music, 99.9." by a quarter inch of feed dust and manure. Static blurred Christmas carols in rhythm with the pulsators. Milking units hung on two Holsteins and a Jersey, each side of the walkway. "Forty percent off the toys your kids really want, at Blain's Farm and Fleet," the commercial interrupted. "Every kiss begins

  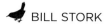 BILL STORK

with Kay; it's not too late to give her something that will shine as brightly as her eyes."

Dave had not spoken a word in two turns of the three units. He turned to his fourteen-year-old son Tommy. With surgical precision, Tommy handed Dave a fresh white dairy towel, in perfect position to wipe the front two teats, and another for the rear. His milking cart aligned squarely on each successive stall divider.

Mental health professionals had designated Tommy so deeply autistic that Dave and Joan should surrender him to an institution, and visit on Sundays. Ten years later, he had yet to miss a milking. Dave never took a towel from the rack not handed by Tommy; and milk testers, truck drivers, neighbors and veterinarians would conjure a feeble excuse to pull on to say "hi" and collect one of Tommy's thunderous hellos and hugs.

The ghost of Hank Williams could have strolled down the barn aisle strumming and moaning "I'm so lonesome I could cry." All Dave could hear was the whistling wind through the barn boards. Drifted snow and chaff were all that covered the floor of the hay mow. Wood stanchions strained as cows stretched for a scrap of silage, their 40-grit tongues licking bare concrete.

Crops that couldn't grow through cracked earth of the dust bowl drought of '88 were stranded by fall rains. If winter snow fell and spring rains came, it would be 6 months before the first mouthful of new green feed.

Christmas is a time for family. To a man of faith, it is the celebration of the birth of Jesus Christ. To a farmer it is the time when he validates the scar on his brow, the hitch in his gait, and the empty seat at the dinner table during silo-filling or calving. Christmas is when he thanks his family for the weddings left early and parties missed.

Any man worth his Red Wings and Carhartts wants more than anything to see his children do a jiggy dance in their footie pajamas in front of the Christmas tree, and to be proud to compare gifts with their friends from town; for his son to have the rechargeable

Air Soft rifle, his daughter the Barbie Jeep and his wife something to adorn her neck or finger and stop the banter cold at volleyball night.

At 45 years old and Norway strong, Dave could cut, split and stack 4 cords of oak before breakfast and mow a thousand bales of hay after lunch. Tonight, forty paces from the barn to the house took all he had. The thought that he would have to stand again was the only thing that kept him from dropping to the packed snow and gravel and curling up like a fetus.

The light of the house poured onto the corner of the porch. Around the tree and hanging from stockings were pairs of socks, gloves and a wooden toy for each boy, wrapped in Sunday's comics. Two three-month-old lab mutts from the neighbor's litter would be Christmas this year. He stood silently and watched Mary and Joe pummel his kindergartener, licking his face and stealing stocking caps.

To a man at rock bottom, all he saw was failure and despair. He looked to the milk house where the "Third Generation Century Farm" plaque hung in the sodium glow of the yard light. He had never imagined it could be the last. Nausea struck with the all-consuming thought of the half-empty bulk tank.

He pried the heel of the rubbers off his work boots and crept into the mud room to hang his coat. There on the shelf was the .357 that sat high out of reach but loaded, for security and varmints. In the space of what could have been minutes or hours he picked it up and put it down a dozen times.

He tried to walk into the light of the kitchen by the family to whom he was the rock. Each time, he wept and gagged. Without a word, he took down the pistol, latched the doors and returned to the cold and dark.

He sat on the porch, forearms across his knees, clutching the cold blue steel. Enveloped in steam as the barn sweat off his waffle weave cotton evaporated into the night, he began to convulse. In one motion he sat bolt upright and pulled the hammer, raised his elbow high and pressed the barrel tight to his temple.

 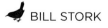 BILL STORK

In a silent primal scream he mashed the trigger, the hammer dropped and the pin fired. The explosion of the hand-held cannon echoed across snow drifts and frozen streams, over Grant County hills and through the valleys; fading to silent over the coal-black waters of the Mississippi.

On impact, 125 grams of lead, traveling 1,500 ft per second, ripped a two-inch gash through two sides of the steel cap... of his concrete silo.

Dave had found himself on the porch with a gun to his head more as the last act of a desperate man, than a product of planning. He had given little thought as to what might lie on "the other side." Whatever he had expected, sprawled in a snowdrift with a sore wrist and a deafening ringing in his ear while having his face washed by a 30 lb lab pup was not it.

As fate would have it, the farmer's lowest point and time of greatest need precisely coincided with Mary's most urgent desire for lovin'. Totally oblivious, or keenly aware, she saw a victim at precisely her level and covered in sweat. There was but one thing to do: knock him down and lick him.

Dave would regain his senses long before his hearing. He staggered into the living room and dismissed his dishevelment, "rough calving." There was no way for the family to know how to react to the ghost in their midst.

After bedtime stories, the boys tucked in, Dave returned to the porch. The Mail Pouch Tobacco thermometer read 8 degrees F. The dampener on the screen door barely kept it from slamming. Each time he opened and let the door fall, it shut and latched securely.

He walked out from under the overhang, looked past the stars into the crystalline sky, nodded and mouthed a silent "Thank You."

He climbed the stairs, crept into the bedroom and pulled Joan close. Crawling under the heirloom quilt, he brushed her long dark hair and kissed her temple. Holding her tighter than he ever had, he slept not a wink.

Rains in the spring of 1989 would quench the parched land and bring feed to the hungry herd.

Tommy eventually committed to an institution: the University of Wisconsin – Platteville. He would graduate with honors and go on to teach Agriculture and Special Education.

Brett, the kindergartener, would be the fourth generation. He and his wife would give Dave and Joan their first grandchild.

Christians, agnostics and animal lovers may debate, but inarguable is that the 50-stanchion, red hip roof dairy where the 5th generation farmer rides the milking cart with his dad and grandpa, would be someone's repurposed barn wood picture frame, were it not for a lab mutt farm dog named Mary.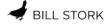

BILL STORK

Norway's Gold

Once every four years, the world comes together for an apolitical celebration of good will and athletic competition. The Winter Olympics entertain and distract us from Super Bowl Sunday through the dregs of February. By closing ceremonies, we are but days away from March Madness, and average daily temperatures near 35F. You can find grown men in coveralls talking to little old ladies about "the Double Lutz" and a "switch nose butter triple cork 1600 double Jeanie" in line at Sentry.

We love the back stories, like how snowboarder Justin Reiter lived out of his Toyota Tundra for a shot at the dream. We fight tears as, after fighting to retain his gold medal in freestyle moguls, Alex Bilodeau embraces his brother and dedicates the victory to him.

"How can I have a bad day? If I'm tired, or it's cold, I take one look at my brother who has cerebral palsy, and go to work."

Advances in nutrition, training and technology push athletes where they have never gone before. As if we were slopeside, we watch images delivered to our TVs from half a world away, generated by digital cameras mounted on drones, hovering above the mountain.

Be as it may, three of the world's so-called "Superpowers" are being taken to task by a country that covers an area slightly bigger than Wisconsin and Illinois combined.

At press time, Norway is in third place with 14 overall medals. Impressive by any count, until you take into account that the "Land of the Midnight Sun" is the second least populous country in all of Europe. Four times more people live in Chicago and suburbs than in all of Norway. If we are to consider medals per capita, then USA and Germany have brought home one piece of hardware for every 19 million residents.

Two-thirds of the way through the games, Norway has already medaled three times for every million Vikings. In the Trondelag region, 8th graders who have yet to win an Olympic medal are made to sit in the back of their classrooms.

I could not be less surprised.

This is not based on the fact that Norwegians are the only people I know who raise tobacco that has to be planted, trimmed, picked and stripped ...by hand. Nor is it because they gather in church dining halls to celebrate cod soaked in lye.

Oslo rests at the same latitude as Anchorage, Alaska, and the only thing they are famous for — other than really long words with precious few vowels — is fjords. It is safe to assume that a young Norseman in search of romance is going to have to ski, skate or climb a mountain any direction he goes. Six months of the year, he'll be doing it in the dark.

With the above points being valid and true within the limits of artistic license, I stand solid in my prediction of Norwegian supremacy in the 2014 Winter Olympics, based on Jim Skaar.

In 1864, the Civil War raged. So consumptive was the effort, that there was a shortage of able-bodied farm hands to raise cattle and grain desperately needed by the country and troops. Delegations were sent to Northern Europe. Norwegians were known to be drawn to farm work and regarded of the highest integrity, industrious and sober. Wisconsin land owners gladly paid $25 to bring Norsemen to Quebec by boat. Trains would complete the passage to Chicago and Milwaukee, where they were hired on the spot.

From there the trail goes cold. Somehow they got to Stoughton, and haven't left yet.

It would be another 128 years before I graduated from veterinary school, by which time Jim Skaar farmed half of eastern Dane County. As advertised, he was of strong mind and stronger body, and he hadn't missed a day of work since he stepped off the train. Sobriety not guaranteed.

If Norwegians ski and skate anything like Jim Skaar farms, the rest of the world is playing for pride. When it comes to tenacity, the "The Screamin' Norwegian" makes a Bulldog look like a Peekapoo.

Nola called to have me look at a cow that had recently freshened. As I approached from the east, I could not help but notice an International sitting motionless in the middle of a field. Early in the

 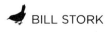 BILL STORK

spring when farmers are looking to clean the cow yards, behind it was a spreader, mounded high and buried to the axle. The frost recently out of the corn stubble, the IH sat spinning helplessly on the grease. Logic might suggest throwing the PTO, dumping a few tons of manure, and driving right out. But leaving a full load of manure in one spot, to be spread once the field was dry, well before planting — Jim Skaar would have nothing of the sort.

He marched a straight line back to the shed, only to return with the heaviest log chain and the biggest piece of equipment on the farm. Lost on a Norwegian in full rage was that, while a Dressen rubber-tired end loader is perfectly suited to load feed, it is as useless as a Toyota Prius for pulling a tractor and spreader out of the mud.

Not to be deterred, in minutes Jim had the end loader hooked to the tractor. Gently pulling slack from the chain, he throttled up. Nothing, not an inch.

As all four wheels started to spin, he dug a hole of his own. Like a beagle on fresh tracks, bound and determined, he backed up. Some of my Dad's more succinct words of wisdom echoed through my head: "If I EVER see you yank on a chain tryin' to pull somebody out, I'll kick your butt 'til your nose bleeds."

With ten feet of a 75 lb log chain lying in the mud, he buried the throttle and let fly.

The chain came taut and snapped. The free end flew through the back window so fast the glass broke in the shape of the chain links flying through it. Before coming to rest around Jim's feet, it grazed the hat on his head and shattered the defrost fan mounted in the upper corner of the windshield. Thankfully this Norseman was blessed with more tenacity than height.

Having finished our cow work, Brian and I stood by the tailgate of my truck. I looked and started to ask, "He wouldn't...." but by then Brian was flyin' across the field.

Unfazed by near decapitation, Jim straightened his Red Man hat, flew through the door and over the catwalk. He had a double square knot tied in the chain and was back on the throttle when Brian jumped into the bucket screamin', wavin' and gasping for breath.

"Good God, you dumb old man, I don't have time to scrub your brains out of this rig before I feed cows tonight."

Days short of his 75th birthday, I pulled on to Skaardal farm. From the machine shop to the calf barn was nothing but elbows and backsides and perpetual motion. A posse of high school farm boys drafted Jim. He'd pause to bark another order and all three would collapse on the nearest hay bale or tailgate.

As I scrubbed my boots and stowed my gear, I asked his wife Nola about the commotion.

"Oh Doc, Jimmy's getting his other knee replaced tomorrow," she explained. "Nothin' doin' but he's gotta get everything done... and NOW."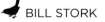

Lights, Camera, Action!

It was inevitable.

Dr. James Alfred Wight graduated from Glasgow Veterinary College in 1939. Absorbed fully by the rigors of practice and parenting, it would take 25 years, several rejections from publishers, and encouragement from his wife before he would put pen to paper and tell the tales of a veterinarian in rural Yorkshire. Half a decade later, his first collection of "little cat and dog stories" (as he modestly referred to them) would make their way to New York City.

For generations to follow, and to this day, James Herriot's "All Creatures Great and Small" is read by millions of animal lovers the world over. Many become veterinarians as well. By 1975, the television series of the same title was wildly popular in both the UK and USA.

Dr. William Stork graduated from the University of Illinois in 1992. Similarly distracted, it would be 20 years before he would begin to chronicle the beauty of rural Wisconsin and the strength of her people on a blog respectfully titled "In Herriot's Shadow." Published in the Lake Mills Leader and Cambridge News, his stories are circulated to hundreds and read by Don Grant and Gary Edmunds. We sincerely appreciate you both.

At the risk of confirming my partner Sheila's suspicions, I use idle time wisely. While slow-driving a tractor load of split oak in order for the sway in the drawbars not to spill the load, and resting my back, I practice pointing and waving. In my mind, I prepare a well-thought response for when the call comes. For reasons not suitable for public discussion, I know what I would have told Oprah. Rather than deal with the rejection, she cancelled her show. I am looking forward to Ellen most, and I fear that in order to appeal to the Jerry Springer audience, I would have to step far outside of the veterinary code of ethics.

Right on schedule, the call that I fully expect to launch my second career came not from Kelly and Michael or Dr. Phil, but from the Watertown Public Access Cable Channel.

Our neighborhood is usually pretty calm, so I was a bit concerned at what commotion might ensue. I had visions of make-up trailers, satellite trucks, production crews, props, sets and lighting. I'm not sure what they do, but every good movie I have seen lists several "grips" in the closing credits. Parking space could be a problem.

I was fully prepared for the director to yell "CUT!" through her megaphone, hop down from her canvas chair, waving and ranting onto the set to correct my posture, gesture and diction. I was sure to show up well rested, properly fed and hydrated. I've seen interviews with Clooney and Pitt, who tell of marathon days on location.

The stars aligned and we met at the clinic on Saturday, February 22nd. One of our favorite clients, Lisa Steffl, hosts a terminally endearing show called "Ask Aunt Ann." Set in the sepia-toned sixties, she fields questions from pickles to pet care.

Lisa arrived with her dachshund, Lucky, and director Jill Nadeau by way of a Honda hybrid, shortly after noon. I surveyed the parking lot and highway V: not a semi to be seen. I assumed that for a first-time actor not to be intimidated, and to maintain the organic feel of the show, it was best to go minimal.

Rather than show my hand, I chose to let my acting chops speak for themselves. I was no stranger to the bright lights and silver screen.

At Christmas break, 1969, Mom took me to our local NBC affiliate WAND-TV, for a taping of "Romper Room." Nearly 40 years before smartphones and Facebook, it was a televised playdate, complete with moms in cat eye glasses and bouffant hairdos. Anyone could be a part of the studio audience, but, as it turned out, participation is by invitation.

I was not a defiant kid by nature, but when they broke out the "stilts" (plastic drink cups with a loop of string attached to hold them to your feet), I could not contain myself. Totally off script came a tall, thin kid with big, red, chef-salad hair, wearing Sears Toughskins and a silk cowboy shirt... right on to the set. I had one foot in and just about to step up when I received a rather unceremonious hook.

 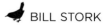 BILL STORK

Ten years before braces, I turned to the camera and smiled right through my great big overbite. I will not tell you it carried a fraction the stigma of having been named "Sue," but "Buck tooth Bill" will put a little gravel in your gut and spit in your eye.

Feeling secure that my previous acting experience would serve me well, I headed in to the taping of "Ask Aunt Ann." The camera was formidable, and made a guy feel authoritative to stand in front of it, like being on location for the ten o'clock news. Regrettably, the battery was dead so the resourceful director mounted her Nikon Sure Shot on the tripod and set it to video.

For a fee of a hundred "Zuke's" treats, Lucky agreed to be our patient. I searched for the blanket that would feature him the best and look good on camera.

Action! Aunt Ann turned to me: a rather forward-thinking viewer had written to ask, "What do we need to know to properly prepare our dogs for warm weather?"

I had seven minutes.

On that day, the wind chill was -14, making it hard to imagine that the first ticks are less than a month away. Retired teachers overwinter in Arizona, Texas and Florida; ticks hunker down under pine bark, needles, dander and leaves. As soon as the snow shrinks away, they are literally out for blood. Mosquitoes won't be too far behind, carrying heartworms far and wide. In order to ensure your pets were not exposed to heartworm disease or Lyme and other tick-borne diseases, last spring through November, it is important for them to be tested yearly, and protected against new exposures.

One of the splendors yet to be realized of winter 2014 is the first short-sleeve day. Every man, woman, child and dog will be outside from dawn 'til dusk. A parent's dream; a vet's fret.

Mike McCarthy would not gather the Green Bay Packers on Sunday morning, and then suit up and play the Chicago Bears that afternoon. It is equally concerning for Leon the labrador to go from couch to dog park, overnight. Our associate, Dr. Deanna Clark, CCRT, points out that during a two mile walk for mom and dad, an off-leash Lassie following her nose will travel a marathon, 26.2 miles.

We have a tendency to assume they will know when to quit. Not so much. Aaron Rodgers could throw balls for a high-drive Jack Russell Terrier until his arm fell off. Those first outings of spring our canine athletes are at their peak weight and least fitness. We see an abundance of knee, hip and shoulder injuries just as the grass turns green.

The injuries that take place under the dog's own power are painful for your pet and expensive for the owner, but carry the best prognosis for return to the field. HBCs (hit by car), HBDB (dune-buggies), HBATV (you get the drift) are much less likely to make it back to the starting lineup, over-represented in the spring, and for the most part, preventable.

I hope to ride the Wright Stuff Century this year on Labor Day Weekend. A winter of writing, watching Olympics and splitting firewood would leave me at war with my saddle if I were to ride farther than the Sentry store this afternoon. If Henry will chase a hundred balls in July, throw twenty for him in March. Think of what would be a normal summer outing, and cut it in fourths.

Be sure and feed several hours before exercise. Don't forget hydration. Most dogs, with the exception of select Schnauzers, have yet to master the valves on Camelback hydration units. Unlike a horse, you can lead a dog to water and get him to drink. Mix a little low-sodium gravy, tuna juice or canned food with a bowl of water an hour before exercise. In order to avoid gastric bloats and torsions, don't allow your dog to tank up when they are in the throes of panting.

If all goes well, we will see another 10 days below zero. In doing so, a few more Lyme-infected ticks lying under your pine trees will die, and we will set a 144-year record for days below zero. When this awesome winter relents, we will celebrate green grass and sunshine like it's 1999. ❧

 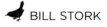 BILL STORK

Little Annie is No Orphan

As veterinarians and animal lovers, our focus follows a fairly predictable curve as we progress through the stages of pets' lives.

With puppies, we talk about crate and toilet training. Through the middle years, our concerns are often skin and ear problems. We focus on feeding the best diets, and on keeping their weight down, their minds engaged and their bodies fit. By the time we have the first decade in the rearview, we are thinking about quality of life and comfort, like glucosamine and anti-inflammatory drugs to diminish the impact of arthritic changes.

In the exam room, we will often lead with a general question, "Any specific problems or concerns?" We've come prepared to address concerns about weight loss, cognitive issues, incontinence and dental health.

I was not prepared for Annie. It's been two weeks, and I may be smiling for two years.

I asked Sheldon about the 14-year-old dog, "How is her energy, appetite, mobility, water consumption?"

He nearly knocked me off my axis, "Is there any way we can slow her down a bit?"

A dramatic difference from our first visit with Annie, two years ago…

The leash hung limp between nine-year-old Ben and his Cocker Spaniel. It has been said that veterinarians are handicapped compared to their human medical colleagues, as our patients can't speak. I beg to differ.

In the back yard Ben ran, jumped and played in fits and starts like Billy from Family Circus. With Annie's leash — more a metaphor than restraint — looped around his wrist and clipped to her collar, he slowed to her pace.

In the clinic lobby, Annie stepped onto the scale in stop-time. First one paw, then another. With her right rear on the scale, she quick-stepped and rocked so that her left could bear the weight. At 11 kilos on the nose, she had lost a third of her body weight.

Plenty aware of the quart of treats six inches from her fully functional, bird dog nose, she hadn't the strength to lift her head or the energy to ask. When our technician, Sheila, opened her palm to offer a freeze-dried liver morsel, she rolled it around her mouth in search of a tooth that didn't hurt. Eventually, she opted to swallow it whole. Her tail feathers swayed as she wagged twice in gratitude.

Her coat was scraggly and coarse. Large patches of her flank were bare. Her skin was mottled and bloody.

As veterinarians we are bound by oath to the "prevention and relief of animal suffering." and to "protect and enhance the human-animal bond."

As humans we are often well served to give our first impressions... a second chance.

The silence and lack of expression from Annie's family spoke volumes. It might take a battery of tests, a small pharmacy and divine intervention, but it was clear we were to stop at nothing to improve the comfort in Annie's remaining years.

Antibiotics would clear the sores on her skin, and careful choice of the right CoxII inhibitor would cease the fire in her knees and hips, while sparing her kidneys. Five tenths of a milligram of Levothyroxine would support her underactive thyroid gland.

Our technicians Megan and Sheila worked with their trademark efficiency. In the 30 minutes from blood draw to «Voila!." we learned how special Annie is to the Parson family.

Memorial Day weekend 2002, Annie was a puppy; Ben was a toddler. Along with two other families, the Parsons had hiked the spectacular East Bluff of Devil's Lake State Park. Ben rode on dad's back, while Annie tested the limits of her leash. No scrap of scat or animal track within six feet of either side of the trail got past the

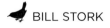 BILL STORK

busy little bird dog on the outbound trek. Nary a chipmunk, grey squirrel, groundhog or white-tail deer escaped her nose or eyes, yet she never so much as yapped.

The expedition stopped for photo ops: pine trees, formation of granite and the ripples of the lake that would find their way onto Christmas cards. They refueled, hydrated and rested their backs. On the return loop, the trail-side banter became muted and sparse with every step closer to the beach shimmering at the foot of the bluff. Annie, having spent her puppy exuberance, was pleased to trot down the trail toward camp.

Their collective "trail sore" was no match for the cool emerald waters of Devil's Lake. Men, women, children and dogs waded, splashed, and swam. Fresh from his nap in dad's backpack, Ben toddled on the end of Sheldon's finger. He punched the water, laughing uproariously as it splashed in his face. In an hour or so, the entourage returned to their camp compound.

As the sun dropped over the West Bluff, the fire crackled and hissed as brats and burgers dripped into the coals. Eight canvas-backed Adirondack camp chairs formed a tight circle around the fire's warmth. There was a satiated pause after their feast. As the conversation was about to turn from "did you see that doe and her twin fawns?" to "remember that day in college when we inflated the giant turtle on top of the big, square, grey house?" there came a commotion from the least likely candidate.

When Annie woofed twice and growled, the group's first concern was disturbing the neighboring campers. As she crescendoed from episodic to insistent, heads turned in collective urgency. After having quietly watched every mammal in Devil's Lake State Park scamper through the underbrush, it was downright absurd that it would be an overturned Rubbermaid storage tote that would offend Annie.

Sheldon leapt from his chair and righted the tub, ripping off the lid. There he found Ben, curled in the fetal position, soaked in sweat, and limp as a ragdoll, having used up the last atom of oxygen trying to escape.

With several deep breaths, Ben let out an epic «Waaah!» that echoed between the bluffs and across the lake. Silence, thought and gratitude prevailed for the remainder of the evening.

Annie slept curled in a ball, perhaps oblivious to the hugs and tears, or possibly fully aware. ⬬

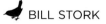 BILL STORK

Get Local

Thanks, Rob

The first Saturday in October the population of Lake Mills grows by 25 percent. People pour off I-94, and sneak in on Hwy 89, by mini-van and SUV with racks and bicycles costing more than my first two cars. Restaurants and gas stations are flooded with aliens seeking carbohydrates, potassium and fluids, sporting tight pants with jerseys that boldly proclaim allegiance to everything from Alma Maters to Wonder Bread.

At 10:00 a.m. they assemble. The Lake Mills Police Department blocks intersections along Highway V as riders flow out of town like the Tour de France, five times bigger and half speed. Last Saturday riders who geared up to endure temperatures in the high 30s and 20mph headwinds were rewarded with more than a barbecue, T-Shirt and free beverages. Wisconsin was in all her glory.

Angry gray clouds made perfect contrast to fiery oaks and maples that lined fields of corn in full harvest. Small children lined the road in Reeseville to high-five riders flying by. After 28 miles of biting headwind we turned on Ghost Hill Road. Miles from anywhere a solitary walker sporting a bright vest and oversized sunglasses pumped his left fist and cheered passing cyclists, as his right hand and white cane rhythmically searched for obstacles. Suddenly, we weren't so cold or tired.

If you have found yourself slowed by traffic or a group riding three abreast, I would ask that you consider a few things. First, be grateful we live in a community where a ten-minute delay is noteworthy. Second, think of your mother, father or family friend who has been assisted by Rainbow Hospice, or perhaps a son, daughter or neighbor who has been treated at UW Children's Hospital.

Tyranena Brewing Company has been a point of pride for our community for nearly 13 years. Offering locals and travelers, farmers and physicians a comfortable place to enjoy expertly crafted and critically acclaimed microbrews, they also give back.

For a decade they have hosted over 1,500 riders for the annual Oktoberfest Bike Ride. Thanks to the generosity of Rob Larson and

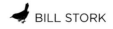 BILL STORK

a herculean effort by Stacey Schraufnagel, with a small army of loyal volunteers, Tyranena has donated over $200,000 to Tomorrow's Hope.

Somehow, that wasn't enough for Rob. So, each November for over 7 years, the Tyranena Beer Run — with 1,400 runners and walkers — has contributed nearly $60,000 and 3.5 tons of food to local food pantries and charities, including the Humane Society of Jefferson County and Rock Lake Activity Center.

Riders and runners come to Lake Mills twice a year to enjoy all our area has to offer. Let us make them feel welcome and recognize the positive impact they and the Tyranena Brewing Company have on deserving local charities. ◀▶

Dairy Month

At 7:30 a.m. on May 17, 2012, all is well at the intersection of Hwy A and Q. A country potpourri of freshly planted ground, alfalfa, and wildflowers floats on a light northwest breeze. Everything is right on schedule for Jefferson County farmers. Tyler Wollin motors up the driveway on his battery-powered John Deere with mom and his yellow lab Maggie. Dressed in plaid shorts, a Gap hoodie and flip-flops, he looks like a 40 lb frat boy, but he's thinking like a farmer.

To grow up on a farm is to be immersed in the virtues of hard work and accountability. For 3-year-old Tyler, it's either a miracle or one of the finest stories of perseverance ever told, because on Sunday, May 31, 1998, all was not well.

At 1:23 a.m., Milford, Wisconsin was hit by a derecho. 111mph straight-line winds ripped the roof off the barn, leveled silos, and nearly broke the spirit of one of the strongest men I know. The Wollin farm was inoperable. Farmers by nature flow to need, and by sunrise the yard was filled with trucks and trailers, and the cows dispersed to three other farms.

Son Erich was a sophomore in college. From growing up on a farm and playing football, he had shoulders like a bull. Yet they were nearly crushed by the weight of a decision: come home to farm and we will build it back... or not.

With Tyler baling hay next to him, what had to be a gut-wrenching leap of faith 14 years ago must seem like serendipity today. It only works by way of bull-dog tenacity, skill and the power of family, and it is not unique.

June is Dairy Month. Please stop to appreciate the men and women who make Wisconsin one of the most beautiful and productive lands in the country, and put food on our tables.

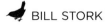 BILL STORK

Claire

Congratulations Claire!

For the precious few of you who don't know Claire Scholten, she knows you. For a year Claire was the smiling voice who greeted you on the phone or at the door of the Lake Mills Veterinary Clinic. There is a good chance she knows your animal's name and medical history, based on your voice.

What you may not know is that each morning she had first milked 50 Jersey cows, fed calves and cleaned the barn with her dad, brother and significant other. On any given day after keeping the peace and flow at the clinic for 8 hours, she would throw off the scrubs, hop back into barn uniform, and do it again.

Baptized with whole, unpasteurized Jersey milk, Claire has grown up immersed in the agricultural mentality. She has shown cattle at every level, and worked in every capacity for several farms. She served as the ultimate ambassador for agriculture in Jefferson County as 2010 Fairest of the Fair.

Most recently, and the accomplishment we salute her for today, she graduated with honors from Lakeshore Technical College Agriculture Short Course, and walked away with the WD Hoard Award for most outstanding student and citizen during the course of the class.

Claire has a deep love for all creatures, great and small, especially Jersey cattle. She has an excellent education base from UW-River Falls, Lakeshore Technical College, and from farming with her father. She has an unquestionable work ethic.

Yet, Claire can't farm.

On her own, that is. A young person today cannot be smart enough, or work hard enough to start farming alone, from scratch. Whether 50 cows or 5,000, never forget the necessity of family.

Today's generation is able to farm as a result of the sacrifice and relentless work of several generations before them, all the while confronted by countless factors out of their control. ◈

Happy Birthday, Ida Behm

Late October in Wisconsin, our rolling fertile fields give way to hay mows that bow to the weight of thousands of bales of alfalfa. Acres of corn, tall as a basketball hoop, turn to bunkers full of silage and fields of stubble.

Sunrise is spectacularly diffracted by bean dust and frost, but now comes far too late to use as a snooze. The horizon will glow but not until you reach the eastbound on-ramp will the first rays remind that you forgot to wash your windshield and to crank the defrost. A quarter year on the calendar past June 21, darkness returns quickly.

It is the time of year when human nature is to cling to the last hope of a T-shirt afternoon. It is also the time when sunset and a subtle error can find a good man clinging to his life.

The front doorbell at the clinic rang for the second to the last time of the day, as Molly the Happy Visla dragged her dad, Ben, out the door into the darkness and on to what's next. The exam room was scrubbed and the lights off to signal day's end. Sheila and Karen wrapped up records and callbacks, while Claire balanced the deposit.

When the door chimed again, no one picked up their head and said "Hi, Ginny." like Norm strolling into Cheers. Sue Nelson blasted into the clinic, dispelling the notion that she was Ginny the cleaning lady, as she flung her "grandma" purse onto the counter.

"Does anyone know what's going on at the corner of B and O?" were her first words.

I was around two corners and half-dressed, but locked ears onto the conversation at once.

Her tone was mono, her eyes creased and her bottom lip quivered. I was intimately familiar with that section of farmland.

"There are floodlights and flashers out in the field, and the Sheriff has the road closed." she reported.

 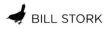 BILL STORK

Finishing the conversion from dog and cat khakis to Pella coveralls in a flash, I dropped everything. I didn't stop to pull on my rubber over-shoes or for the glow plugs to warm the diesel. I cranked the old truck twice and lurched out the parking lot in a cloud of blue smoke. In stony silence, I headed west around the lake and out Hwy B. Officer Delaney would just have to understand.

For those looking to get a bit closer than the refrigerator to the source of their milk, cheese and butter, there is no better place than the Ritchie Behm Farm. From the house he was born in, across a blacktop pad to the hip-roof, half wooden and metal stanchion, basement barn, his commute has remained the same since the day he graduated high school. For that matter, well before. He has hosted guests from a dozen states and six foreign countries.

Ritchie and his mother Ida, have seldom left.

At least once a week, just as I'm pouring Lucky Charms into the leftover milk from my Cornflakes and turning from the "hard news" on the front page to the advice column, the phone will ring.

"This is Ritch Behm," she says.

As if I had suffered complete and catastrophic amnesia overnight, and was struggling to hear the phone over the din of a heavy metal concert at 4:50 a.m., she repeats, "THIS IS RITCH BEHM, B-E-H-M, Highway O, Waterloo."

As if it were not burned on my hard drive, she repeats the telephone number, "8-6-7-5-3-0-9." just as firmly.

"I have a cow under the weather when you have a chance," she finishes softly.

The debate as to turn right at the top of the drive or left is no more. Rather than pump my pecs and learn about President Obama's daily idiocy on Fox News (fair and balanced) at the Lakers Athletic Club, I'll head to the farm. I finish the article in the *Wall Street Journal*, of which I understand a fraction, but somehow feel more sophisticated as a result. I wash my bowl, feed horses, carefully decant a hot pot of Yuban and arrive well before 6:00.

It took at least a half-dozen visits to the Behm farm before I didn't drop my stainless-steel bucket on the concrete and burn a path back to the safety of the 3/4-ton Dodge. Drowning out the milk pump, fans and running water comes a booming, "GET OUT THE DOOR!"

Milked and fed, the first shift of cows do as they are told, and saunter out the door to the silage in the bunk. Stooped by nearly 80 years of farming, cooking, cleaning, raising children, grandchildren and osteoporosis, the diminutive bullhorn shuffles into the milk house. Scarf tied under her chin, and crocs scuffling the lime on the concrete, she feigns surprise, "Oh, you're up already?"

As if I'm not already feeling feeble by comparison. "What'd you bring me for breakfast?" I swear someday I have to take her a hot muffin.

My meandering thoughts coalesced into concern as I turned left onto Hwy O and slowed. Just as the stubble met the corn was a semi-circle of fire trucks and first responders lit up like Friday Night Lights. I swallowed hard and cracked the window for fresh air. The Behm farm has hosted visitors from all over the globe, but technology was somewhere between Olde World Wisconsin and Farm Progress Days.

Silage was picked and chopped by a two-row pull-behind called a Uni. Powered by the tractor that pulled it, there were no shortage of U-joints, PTO shafts, conveyors and teeth to pull a tired man in loose clothing to peril.

Just outside the glow, the med-flight copter sat silent.

There was clearly no need for a veterinarian in the corn field, so I parked in front of the milk house and tore through the door. I was not the first, or the last.

She stood motionless, leaning on the bent rusty gate, and staring into the field through the gap in the barn door. Amber and red flashing lights from the fire engines surrounding the corn-picker strobed her face.

 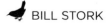 BILL STORK

Eventually there came a singular tear that pulled a rivulet of mascara through the creases in her cheek, and clumped in the lime at her feet. Oblivious to the crowd building behind her she whispered, "I changed that boy's diapers."

Neighbors, friends and a young man: "I was down at the Kroghville Oasis having a beer; my girlfriend's brother used to milk here, and I saw the lights. I milk cows on another farm, how can I help?" he stood as ready to wrestle a bear as milk a herd of cows.

Able-bodied but feebly minded, we all shuffled like so many stooges looking to grab something with a handle, but not sure what to do next.

True to form, Ida made a four-point turn to address the gathering throng, as if she'd expected every last one of us. "WELL, THESE COWS DON'T MILK THEMSELVES, WHO KNOWS HOW TO DO WHAT?"

Rather than wait for an answer, "Good, now let's do it."

Order was restored but not without one last shock as her son Ritchie, a man of 50 whose diapers she had surely changed, and who was assumed to be caught in the jaws of the corn picker, strode into the barn.

Ida's kid brother, "Uncle Phil" had spent the day on the farm helping with fall chores and had stopped to unclog the corn picker. Fortunately, on this day, a farm accident would claim flesh and blood, but not a life. He would lose part of a foot and a hand, and be relegated from organist and vocalist to tambourine at the altar on Sunday mornings. The phantom pains in his missing limbs were unable to mute his spirit and soul.

Whether consciously or not, we are prone to looking for heroes. Basketball stars and bike riders will leave us cherry-picking their attributes and making excuses. On a dairy farm on County Highway O lives a woman who stands a tad over five feet tall and weighs a buck twenty, yet she has the strength of ten thousand men. Ida hasn't had a dozen good night's sleep in her 80 years, yet she's raised five children, a brother and a grandson. Two decades after the heartiest have retired, she cooks, cleans, feeds calves, scrapes barn floors and herds cows. She doesn't know how not to. She is the family and town historian. Neighbors, family and friends take turns in the crosshairs of her sarcasm.

This piece was originally written for her 80th birthday. She is now 82 and slowed only a bit. I think of her every day I put my feet on the floor, and my right ankle and left shoulder ache, and it takes a dozen steps to straighten my back. Ida Behm is, and always will be, a living, breathing source of strength and inspiration. ⬺

 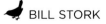 BILL STORK

This Land IS Your Land

I've been to some of the prettiest places on the planet. Thanks to my friends at Lizard Head Cycling Guides, I have pedaled the Continental Divide through Colorado, the canyon country of Utah, and the White Mountains of New Hampshire. That said, I have yet to see a land that can match the muscularity, productivity, fertility and sheer natural beauty of Jefferson County, Wisconsin, at sunrise.

If you take your kids straight to school or throw down breakfast on the I-94 West ramp, please pick a day, set your alarm and take a detour. A cool, clear morning following a warm day works best, at about 6:15. Along Highway Q, between Jefferson and Lake Mills, or along Newville Road, the sunrise fog will hang in layers thin as bedsheets. 150 feet above the drumlins it blankets, the fog diffracts the rays of the sun as it breaks through the trees.

This time of year, the last crop of hay lies flat and fragrant, waiting to be raked, tedded and baled. Slow grazing cattle stand like silhouettes in a diorama, next to hip-roof barns and concrete silos, waiting to be milked.

Kids aren't obligated to appreciate the September sunrise; they will when they're 30. However, it behooves each of us to stop the minivan and recall what these same fields looked like 75 days ago. No dew, no fog — just brown, dead and ugly. It is by the grace of God that enough rain came, in time to yield the crops that surround you, though a fraction of what was expected. It is by technology, tenacity and creativity that our farmers are able to ensure that there will be food on our tables. ❧

It's Definitely About the Bike

I Think I Can

Between appointments on a recent rainy Friday, our receptionist, Claire, commented on a photo.

"It's none of my business," (which has never slowed her before), "but you look as if you are in pain in those pictures. Isn't that supposed to be your vacation?"

I smiled. The first time I went biking in the mountains I was hoping for a few good pictures and a week off. I returned with 250 digital photographs, a whole new perspective, and a brother.

What we call biking trails were carved hundreds of years ago by migrating cattle and Native Americans. They wind like ribbons to the sky. First they climb, seemingly without mercy. Then they traverse, allowing your oxygen-starved mind to behold the Majesty from two miles high. When the snow melts in May and the torrential rains come in August, the water drains peacefully from the trail, preventing erosion and preserving the fragile mountain tundra.

Our days were patterned. Before sunrise, a guide with three days' growth began beating a pan, bellowing COFFEE! After an obligatory trip to the groover and breakfast, we would pack a lunch and break camp. A day of expedition mountain biking requires a few things: 6-10,000 calories, 2,400 mg of Ibuprofen and a handful of Chamois Butter. Without fail, the first several hours of each day are spent climbing. The splendors defy description: from herds of elk to high mountain lakes and streams.

The reward is lunch at the top of the world, devouring roast beef on sourdough, looking down through the clouds at neighboring mountain ranges, all the while gearing up for the monsoon that will soon consume the mountain and its guests.

Skilled guides, campfires, and dueling Dutch Ovens made evening's meal a mile-high feast. Four-year-old cheddar, 10-year-old Scotch, and brand new friends made every night a back country celebration.

Critical Thursday found us camping at "The Vortex." Four days closer to Durango, we were stronger, sharper, and prepared for the Hermosa Creek Singletrack.

In "guide speak" the trip so far had been epic. The next day would be defining.

19 miles and 2,500 vertical feet on the Hermosa Creek Singletrack will leave your senses in overdrive. The trail has its genesis as raging whitewater relaxes into a fertile mountain valley. At times the track is little more than a granite shelf on the canyon wall as she climbs toward the Durango Plateau. Switchbacks, creek crossings and footbridges challenge bike handling skills and resolve as riders part giant ferns that overhang the trail. Glasses fog and nostrils flare, saturated with mountain mist, aspen and pine.

Three hours and one cliffhanger find our expedition at the foot of "the beast." A dozen off-camber switchbacks, thrown into 25% grades; five hundred yards of water bars, roots and rocks are the last obstacle to our first hot shower and mattress in a week.

John Humphries, the man who has become my brother, goes up first. His gloved right hand punches the cobalt sky with a rallying "yeeha!." as he disappears around the first switchback. The idea of climbing this monster from bottom to top was unthinkable, but I wasn't going home with anything left in my tank. I took one last pull of water, clipped in and shoved off.

Switchback number three found me nauseous and honking like a goose. Number four, then five, then six became my goal: the point where I would give up and walk. Having lost the strength to lift my head, by number eight I could never make it to another switchback. I begged my legs for 50 more turns of the crank, then 25, then 10. In minutes that seemed like hours, the final gut-wrenching 180-degree turn loomed. My mind was renegotiating with my body for every turn of the crank. That's when I heard John.

The maniacal Steeler fan was straddling the trail, clenched and growling like Terry Bradshaw in Super Bowl X, "Big man of the Dairyland... YOU WILL NOT QUIT!" I had my orders. In granny low, every stroke buys 13 inches of trail. With my 500th "last." I

 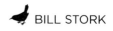 BILL STORK

heaved my front tire over the summit. As I started to fade, John grabbed my seat post and hurled me over the top.

The fitness gained on that trip is long gone; the strength I learned will build for a lifetime. The Hermosa Creek Singletrack is one of the most beautiful places on the planet and an awesome metaphor for life. Whether professional, personal or physical, you will be challenged. We owe it to ourselves, our children and anyone who depends on us to dig deep. If getting from one sunrise to the next seems impossible, get from bed to breakfast. Every step will lend strength to the next. If you find yourself at a place that feels like failure, embrace it as an opportunity to grow. Search the furthest reaches of your mind, body and soul. You will get through.

—◦O◦—

Important postlude that is absolutely true: *I returned to the Hermosa Creek Singletrack several years later. John gathered a different group of riders for hydration and a snack. I was tracing the trail map with my finger and brow creased. "What you lookin' for, Bro?" "Just trying to see how much longer until we get to The Beast." The corners of his eyes wrinkled behind his riding glasses and he wrapped his arm around my shoulder, "About a mile and a half ago."*

—◦O◦—

About the "Groover"

One of the unwavering rules of the mountains is to at least "leave no trace." Ideally we seek to leave things more pristine than we found them, if that is possible. As you can imagine, 10 guests and two guides on the trail for a week, riding for eight hours a day and consuming upwards of 10,000 calories are in serious danger of leaving traces.

Guides are famous for a number of things. They are master mechanics, mountaineers, chefs, storytellers, photographers and EMTs. They are at least as frugal as they are functional. So, when it comes to packing in and packing out you need the perfect vessel for hauling waste miles down treacherous mountain roads. Enter the WWII camo green ammunition box: bulletproof, waterproof, with a securely locking lid; available at any surplus store or flea market for a few dollars each.

By now (if not sooner) the origin of the "Groover" has come clearly into focus. The extent to which the term is literal is dependent on a number of variables. The placement of the groover, the balance, height, weight and strength of the biker also factor into the depth of the situation. Experienced and accurate users are sometimes able to hover.

Adventure travel is all about service and the experience. The guides of Western Spirit Cycling Adventure are masters of their craft. After having described the structure of the facilities, it is the last thing campers will talk about when they return home. Every camera will have five pictures that may be made into a collage and titled, "Views from the Groover." It will be situated in a mountain meadow surrounded by wildflowers, at the edge of a cliff with 180-degree views, or next to a waterfall.

A mountain trip is no place for modesty. Changing rooms are a mat of pine boughs in front of your tent. However, elimination is not flattering for anyone. In the name of privacy and GI motility, there is a system. Curtains and doors would be cumbersome, and obstruct the pristine mountainside. The "key" to the groover is Charmin on the Shifter — a role of TP is hung on the gear shift of the "Trail Boss," the truck that sags our gear up and down the mountain roads, meeting us at the next camp site.

At rush hour, after the cowboy coffee starts to hit bottom, the system breaks down. Those who have been relieved may round the hill to a gauntlet of campers pacing and making small talk. Instead of making it back to the truck, the shrinking roll may be more like a baton in an Olympic relay.

It is worthy of note that in the decade since my first trip, the groover has gone through as many upgrades as the I-phone, with a fraction of the fanfare. Recent models have come to incorporate both a lid and a seat. The views? Just as spectacular. ⬬

BILL STORK

Mbeep, Beep! What's Up, Doc?

I've just returned from a cycling trip through the remotest deserts and canyons of Southwest Utah.

To try and comprehend the effect of thousands of years of water on sandstone is mind-numbing. A lone rider on a ribbon of tortuous blacktop snaking through the red and white sandstone canyons, buttes and mesas is microscopic. Indeed, a cloud of dust, a cartoon bird and an anvil falling on an unsuspecting coyote's head would not have been a surprise, especially as the miles ground on and dehydration and hypoglycemia set in.

Typically, 50 or so miles into our 70-mile days, the head would get heavy and vision would narrow. It was then that I would start to appreciate what was taking place on the desert floor. Like a string section behind an opera's tenor, the yellow rabbit brush and pale green sage contrasted the red sand, and slowed and divided the occasional torrential rain. Near the confluence of mostly dry river beds, stems turned woody and leaves turned gold — an outright delight to the 'Lucky 13', guests of Lizard Head Cycling Guides.

The physical beauty of this barren land is moving. However, it was the acquaintance of a 78-year-old, retired cardiac surgeon that proved to be humbling, and inspirational.

A sliver on the horizon, not necessarily traveling in a straight line, but always moving, the rider would eventually come into focus. Rick, 32 years my senior and having ridden a bike for exactly two years, started a short while before the rest of the group, traveled every inch of tortuous blacktop, and finished each ride while we were savoring our first recovery drink (beer).

Each morning with Lizard Head Cycling Guides starts with a spectacular meal at a unique restaurant. Breakfast is followed by a day of riding and hiking the most spectacular roads and trails one can imagine with a group of diverse and interesting people. We ride at least a metric century, climbing nearly a vertical mile per day, in whatever weather may fall from the sky.

Day 5 was nothing short of epic. We began at Slot Canyon Inn, Escalante Utah. It was impossible not to stop at the Keva Coffee House for espresso before rolling to the trailhead at Calf Creek at the foot of Hell's Backbone. Water in the desert is a commodity, so when a rushing river fuels a bed of green in the floor of a canyon, it is well worth the hike to find its origin. In this case, it must have been from heaven, as our three-mile hike terminated at a 150- foot waterfall pouring from the rocks above. It was there in the cool mist that I sat down to talk to Rick.

After watching him all week, gracious and thankful, I asked if he had a separate personality in the operating room. He had laid down his scalpel only three months previous. This man had spent a 40-year career repairing defects in the hearts of newborns and bypassing occluded arteries in the hearts of parents and grandparents. Preserving quality of life is the kind of thing that could give a person a bit of an ego. His response was simple,

"First, Bill, my skills are no greater than the people who cleared the ground and built our hospitals, and I am of no value without those who assist me. Secondly, it is not a gift, it is a privilege." ◈

BILL STORK

Miles and Miles of Texas

Only a few minutes ago, the forest floors and roadsides of Wisconsin exploded with the colors and perfume of spring wildflowers. Yet, in just a few weeks, most of us will gather to feast and give thanks.

I am fortunate in many ways, not the least of which is to have a family solid and supportive as bedrock and a stable of amazing friends. Some are so profound as to tint and focus the lens through which I view the world; none more so than John Humphries.

John is a gluten-free, organic, leave no trace, tree-hugging man of the mountains. He owns a company called Lizard Head Cycling Guides. His energy and passion could make a 40-mile ride from Rockford to Beloit epic, but he tours groups through some of the most barren and beautiful roads on planet Earth, resting at oases plush, unexpected and out of place, capable of melting 100 miles of road weariness and saddle soreness in 15 minutes.

Each year I wait for John to tell me at which airport to meet him; the details will fall into place. For 15 seasons we have ridden through mountain passes, valleys and the deserts of Colorado, Utah, Arizona and New Mexico. I have toted bags, loaded bikes, built fires and bided time.

On August 15, 2013, he called.

"Bill, I am taking a trip through the hill country of Texas. It's a small group, I'm short- handed, and I need another guide."

I tried to remain cool, all the while feeling like Seneca Wallace on Monday Night Football when Aaron Rodgers went down.

I was qualified and confident. Driving a truck and backing a trailer are second nature. I can cook Dutch oven ribs in a monsoon or fix a flat, and, most importantly, I work cheap.

As we have come to expect from Lizard Head Cycling guides, aka John Humphries, the trip was spectacular. The hill country is a unique, stark and spectacular piece of the great Republic of Texas. Topographically rugged, and famous for its limestone shelf, water is sparse and the entire 25-county region has less top soil than a community garden on the east side of Madison.

May through September the climate is roughly equivalent to the inside of a zip-lock bag at night. The region was occupied in the mid-1800s by bands of ferociously independent English, Irish, Germans and Czechs looking to escape the oppression of their home land, but not until they wrestled it away from the Apaches and Comanches.

Day 1, I drove the Mother Ship. She's a one-ton Ford passenger van, pulling a 22ft enclosed trailer heavily loaded with all the comforts of home. The whole rig is emblazoned with a half dozen 4-foot images of the sun rising over the iconic Lizard Head Pass near Telluride, Colorado, framed by a bike wheel.

With hazards flashing and "CAUTION: BIKE TOUR AHEAD" across the end gates, we wound through the ranch roads. Blend into our surroundings, we did not. My job was to ensure the riders were hydrated, fed and safe, and to keep the boss updated on the Pittsburgh Steelers vs. Oakland Raiders score.

Day 2 was my first day on the bike. We roamed ranches, over cattle guards, through riverbeds and past wineries and orchards, pausing to watch a half-dozen antelope run past a charging herd of whitetail deer, resembling a crotch-rocket passing a motor scooter. Later, I called my dad to tell him I had truly found the land, "where the deer and the antelope play." Eighty miles south of Austin, and a million miles from civilization, there was little wonder how this land came to be the identity of characters from Lyndon B. Johnson to Willie Nelson.

Noon on Monday brought us to the intersection of Waring-Welfare Road and Farm to Market 1621. Waring, Texas inhabits four blocks; population 59. Downtown consists of a post office, zip code 78074, and the General Store, famous for its Wednesday night steak fry.

Across from the General Store was a welding and machine shop, with a two-table diner on the front corner.

The screen door banged shut as I paused to adjust from the midday glare to the dingy confines. Well before I could see, there came

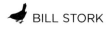

a hearty, "Howdy," as if they had been expecting a 6'4" praying mantis in Velcro tap shoes, Lycra shorts, and a faded Chili Pepper do-rag at any moment. In time, my pupils dilated and I could see the greeting came from the mechanic, having coffee with a cowboy.

My native tongue can only be described as "central Illinois mush-mouth." 21 years in Wisconsin has tempered that with an occasional hard Germanic consonant, and a few rounded Os. 48 hours in Texas will leave anyone with a soft drawl. "Goood Mornin'," I replied.

"What can we do for y'all?" the mechanic asked, though there was only one of me.

There was a little cooler with a glass door and rotating shelves sitting in the corner. "Well if I could talk you out of that last piece of chocolate pie, that would be great. You might just be the guys who could answer a couple of questions I had."

Here in Wisconsin, I would not hesitate for a minute to use "y'all," "reckon," and "fellas." At J and S Machine Shop and Diner, talking to a cowboy and a mechanic, it seemed contrived.

I was fascinated by the man-made "tanks" used to contain the flash floods and water the cattle. I was interested in the goat and fine-wool market suited to the sparse landscape of central Texas. The one thing I had not been able to figure out were some of the fences: at times 8-10 feet tall, woven wire with steel posts and cross members, they were Folsum State Penitentiary issue, minus the razor wire.

I had to ask, "Do y'all have goats down here with 12-foot vertical leaps?"

Chuckling politely, he replied, "Naw, but the hand-raised trophy bucks and bull elk do. Rich folks from Austin and Dallas pay $30,000 to come out and hunt for the weekend."

Before leaving, I asked the cowboy about his operation. He ran a Brahman cross cow calf operation and raised crops. I asked how many head of cattle.

"'Nuff to eat ma feed," with a grin barely perceptible under the brim of his white Resistol.

Knowing the answer, but unable to resist, I asked how much crop land.

"'Nuff to feed the cattle."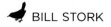

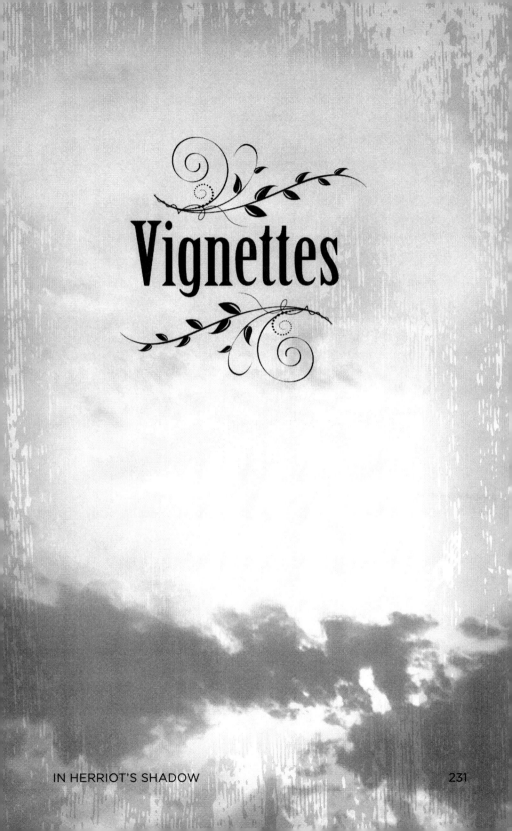

Vignettes

Nine Below Zero

Ain't this a pity people, ain't this a cryin shame,
Well it's nine below zero, she put me down for another man
– Mckinley Morganfield aka Muddy Waters

With a foot of "lake effect" snow and the "Windy City" earning its doubly-intended moniker for the day, Anita was profoundly concerned that a trench coat, rubbers and wool hat would not be enough to get Kish to the "L" station. Van singing "Caravan" through the hidden wires of his IPod would transport his soul to a warmer clime.

On the same day here in Wisconsin, I turned down Holzheuter Lane to the Haack farm to attend a sick cow. I cradled the wheel and mashed the accelerator. The Cummins Diesel punched through a hood-high drift that rolled over the windshield like a wind tunnel. I kicked the barn door free and flung myself into the vestibule and out of the wind. An LB White propane heater hung from a pair of old calving chains, pumping heat into the parlor like an eyedropper in the ocean.

Ryan with a 5-foot pry bar, and Pete with a 16-pound sledge stand knee deep in the gutter, doing battle with a frozen barn cleaner while sporting "grey" water facials. Just short of noon, Ryan is starting his second eight-hour day and Pete is still in his muck boots and rubber elbow-length gloves from third shift at Oscar Mayer.

From Ace Hardware to the Kwik Trip, "Merry Christmas" and "Fare thee well" have been supplanted by "STAY WARM." As if "life-threatening wind chill" and "arctic blast" doesn't get our attention, meteorologists use freshly minted terminology like "polar vortex" to accentuate the severity of the conditions.

As a practicing Catholic and cafeteria Buddhist, might I suggest that we become one with, if not celebrate the beauty of, the "polar vortex."

It's fun just to say, but there are precious few opportunities to truly "hunker down."

 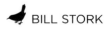 BILL STORK

It may be so simple as to buy milk, water and bread. For those outside the city limits with "W" or "N" before their fire numbers, there will be chipping ice, opening water tanks and securing wind breaks to protect the horses and cattle. We stack wood in the end loader and pile it in the garage until there is enough to last until the weather breaks. The steel handle of the splittin' maul sinks the heat from our hands and we drum up images of the pioneers who came to this land 150 years ago. Any notion of kinship fades with the reality that the wood they burned was not for ambiance, but their only source of heat. They did not have a chainsaw, or a tractor to haul it and it was long before polypropylene, smart wool and fleece.

Contrary to our personal preferences, we need this weather. Majestic mountain forests of Colorado have been decimated, Wisconsin is stepping up laws to prevent the movement of fire wood and there have been years when the prevalence of Lyme disease in Northern Wisconsin has approached 30%. Let's just see how the Pine Bark Beetle, Emerald Ash Borer and Deer Tick like 48 hours of 20 below zero.

Wise men, namely Ryan Haack, have theorized that the anticipation is harsher than the reality. When the day arrives, you find yourself dumping down to survival mode. Knowing that your bare hand budget is at an all-time low, you pocket your leatherman in the "ready" position before leaving the milk house. You haul bales and turn your back to the wind. In one smooth motion you bury the gloved hand in your armpit, grab the tool, cut the twines, stow it and return to the glove. As quickly as possible you return to the dashboard of the truck your second pair of gloves.

A 2-foot glacier surrounding a cow tank and a pick axe are your best friends. Ten minutes of breaking and hauling ice, and your hands will stay warm long enough to set an IV needle and treat a cow for ketosis.

If there is a single reason to not trade ten below for a white sand beach and a rum drink with an umbrella... it is the brotherhood. At two a.m. in a white out you're are not headed to the Redbox to rent

"The Titanic." The lights in the distance are a county truck plowing and salting, a milk truck, tow truck, plumber or a line crew. You give as much of where you think the center line is and still stay on the high side of the ditch. Staring hard at the tracks you're riding, you clench your jaw and speak a quiet "git 'er done" to the empty cab.

As if you need any more reason to celebrate the weather we just endured, I offer 10:48 a.m., January 9th. I passed Dave Schroeder's grain bins at 5:30 Monday morning January 6, my truck read -18F. Temperatures were to remain stubbornly below zero for most of the week. Four days later I passed Dave's bins and it was -16. I was unfazed. I palpated a half- dozen cows at Gene Mess', and it was "up" to -12. A quarter mile and 20 minutes later at Tim Claas' -10. By mid-morning at the Haack farm Ryan and I still had to slow our pace, as to not generate wind chill.

In the space of eight miles and the ten minutes it took to drive from Oak Park Rd. to our home on Hwy 18, the temperature rose to 16 degrees F. Yellow boots, green coveralls and stocking hat, I spread my arms wide to absorb the splendor and did a little dance, right there in the driveway.

To be certain there are those for whom this weather is a true hardship. The price of LP Gas has tripled in 6 weeks. With thermostat set at 60, the furnace blows warm air and an impending sense of despair. Worse yet, there are those who have no furnace, no food, and no hope. ❧

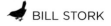 BILL STORK

Rough Rider

I consider myself fortunate in more ways than I could count. One of the greatest is to have a number of friends who are role models. My friend Scott Clewis is learned, well-dressed, well-spoken, and prone to breaking into spontaneous lectures. Given that I usually learn something, and couldn't get a word in anyway, I listen.

Scott's most recent diatribe was on our 26th President, Teddy Roosevelt. If I had ever known, I had forgotten that the Rough Rider was a man of many talents. He was fluent in five languages, made significant contributions to science, boxed, wrestled, and big game hunted. According to Mr. Clewis, he single handedly dug the Panama Canal with a shovel, but Scott has been known to embellish.

His closing statement was something to the effect of, "they just don't make 'em like that anymore."

Mr. Clewis, I object.

Scott lives in downtown Chicago, and probably doesn't know a single farmer, who, with no fewer skills and shoulders as broad as Mr. Roosevelt, put food on all our tables, against impossible odds.

After a lifetime of working with people and animals, I have a theory that "people kind to animals are inherently good."

This is true of our town. There are business people who choose to share their expertise and energy for the betterment of Main Street, Lake Mills. Men and women with full-time jobs and families take time to mentor and serve as role models. Our teachers have open doors, and sometimes a spot at the kitchen table to help a struggling student.

I am moved by older adults who return home to assist aging parents, spouses who aid failing loved ones, and my Dad. Visiting nurses not only serve as company, but also assist people who otherwise would not be able to live in their homes.

Few have books written about them, and even fewer appear in PBS documentaries. But for those they affect, they are no less heroic.

This Land Was Your Land

July 4th is the day we celebrate our country's independence from Great Britain, and the birth of Democracy.

That may have been true in 1776; it is no more. There is a website where you can watch our trade deficit, in real time. Millions of dollars fly by faster than second hands on a clock. Our national debt is staggering, and the percentage of our country that is domestically owned is diminishing rapidly.

We look to our leaders for a solution. Regrettably, Barack Obama can't help, nor will the next President. You and I, on the other hand, can. There will be no real recovery until this country is once again manufacturing stuff, and people are buying that stuff.

Studies suggest that if each consuming American were to divert $60 per month from imported to domestic products, the result would be 600,000 jobs --- in one year. Even if someone pulled that number from their anatomic posterior, even if it is half true, that is a lot of people working again.

So, what if we made everything here?

To think we can shift the base of manufacturing is dramatically oversimplified. Just as some of Dave Schroeder's corn may end up in a bowl in South America, it will always be less expensive to manufacture electronics in China. Experts like Kishan Khemani, VP and Sr. Consultant for A.T. Kearney feel our return to real prosperity will be by way of innovation.

That said, our every Google search, download and credit card purchase is monitored. That information is used to determine everything from life insurance rates, to how long skirts should be next summer.

We live in a consumer-driven society. Domestically manufactured products are shelved side-by-side with ones made overseas; please look for them. Websites make it easy to order American-made products. Search them.

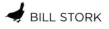 BILL STORK

Buying American-made products requires thoughtfulness. While contemplating the lowest cost of a purchase, think of possibly putting your neighbor back to work. Buying domestic is neither easy nor straightforward. But...

We live in a society where we can sell holey foam rubber shoes to everyone from Joe the Plumber to Doug the Surgeon.

Catchphrases like "how's that workin' for you" spread from the ranches of Wyoming to downtown Chicago in days.

There were 170 million votes for the last American Idol finalists.

Why can't we start a trend that could put people back to work?

Marketing geniuses can anticipate or create a trend, and put products on the shelf in the time it takes to drive from coast to coast. We have been told for decades we can't afford to make things here at home. I say we can't afford to pay someone else to make them while our neighbor is unemployed.

It costs more to manufacture and transport goods made overseas. It is hard for me to believe that in a world where if I buy one suit, I can get two free, there isn't margin left over to make those suits next to the cotton field in Mississippi.

If we the people are suddenly making purchases based on the area code where things are created, industry can respond. ⬦

I Can't

Sunday September 7, 2008, minutes before 7:00 am. Void of fat, their bodies buoyed and insulated by neoprene suits, eyes protected by green and amber polycarbonate lenses, arms and legs marked '1' through '2081' in black grease pencil, they stretch, focus and fend off nausea in the shadow of the Monona Terrace Convention Center. Children, spouses and partners huddle and murmur on the shoreline. Course marshals and guards on stand-up paddle boards stroll through fog that splits the rising sun. AC/DC blasting from concert speakers rips the silence like a 120db alarm clock.

The crack of a starter's pistol echoes off the lake. In an instant, silent anticipation becomes organized chaos in motion. Waves of athletes run six steps and dive. The elite knife through the glass calm lake; the survivors frantically paddle through the chop, fighting for space. Crews on shore clang cow-bells, beat drums and blast air horns.

After 2.4 miles and more than an hour in the water, they stagger and emerge back to dry land. They sprint up the exit ramp of the parking garage, trade neoprene for lycra and fly down the entrance ramp on bikes costing thousands, specifically designed to minimize drag, maximize comfort and to preserve the muscle group required next. And so begins a 112-mile pedal powered tour of America's Dairyland.

Twelve hours, 140.4 miles (and 10,000 calories) later, in the shadow of the state capitol in the now setting sun, they stagger. Like a slow-motion herd of Zombies, in high-tech, wicking fabric by Nike and Under Armor, they round the corner from East Mifflin onto North Pinckney, only a few hundred yards from surviving the 2008 Ford Ironman Classic. The gauntlet on the curbs who love and support them pump their fists and growl, "You can do it, you're almost there!" After 12 hours and 140.4 miles, there's no strength to acknowledge.

Then came bib number 614... long-sleeved, button-up shirt, with a collar.

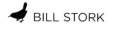 BILL STORK

He had already passed, so we sucked in a lungful, cupped our hands, and let fly "Go, Ryan Haack!" Head lifted, his ears perked as he located the source of support. Fists clenched, with full strides, he wove through the zombies like they were would-be tacklers on a touchdown run, upstream across two lanes of traffic.

"Paige, Calvin, Bill, thanks for coming," he high-fived us and sprinted to the finish. Weighing in at a buck fifty and standing 5'8, Ryan is not physically imposing. However with forearms like a firefighter and hands like a logger, you check to make sure everything is still attached after a high five or a handshake, Ironman or no.

To finish an Ironman competition is a tattoo-worthy accomplishment for anyone who crosses the finish line, or collapses trying. Most work for months to prepare, adhering to prescribed training and diet regimes, often supported by groups, coaches and sponsors. Ryan, on the other hand, can be found in the milking parlor of his family farm by 4:30 every morning, often striding into the darkness for a 17-mile training run when he is finished, if all goes well, by 9:00 p.m.

Worthy of note is that the Ironman is not Ryan's greatest or only athletic endeavor. He has finished a 100-mile cross country race. In Alaska. In February. He prepared by dragging 70 lb log chains across plowed fields. He finished first in the 30-and-over group at the Minneapolis Warrior Dash, among nearly 1,000 others, after milking 120 cows, running 17 miles and driving 4-1/2 hours, the same day.

Worthy of even greater note is that his athletic prowess is not what defines Ryan. Though 24,000 cars travel I-94 in clear view of the farm, and countless planes fly over each day, nothing gets past Ryan. Anchored to the farm, working 80-100 hours a week, he is driven by one of the most open and fertile minds I've ever known. And, until the United States Anti-Doping Administration (USADA) outlaws tall stacks of pancakes, beef sticks and whole milk, he operates definitively in the absence of Performance Enhancing Drugs. In doing so, he has singlehandedly laid waste to the oft uttered yet debilitating phrase, "I Can't."

History will show that the worship of heroes will frequently find us disappointed, or sorting. The good news is that if we are looking for motivation and inspiration, we can often look to the other side of our dining room table, the friend at the next desk, or in a 12-cow flat barn parlor, at the end of Holzeuter Lane.

*** *As I waxed poetic of the value of hard work and the merits of a farm lifestyle, my son Calvin shattered the bliss, "Dad if Ryan had so much energy, why hadn't he passed the Zombies?" I could only speculate, but the numbers later showed that the answer, my friend, is in the swim. It has been said by seasoned triathletes, "Ryan, I have never seen a human spend so much energy, and move forward less, than you in the water." Of 2081 swimmers, he finished in 2016th place. With half the population of Lake Mills, Wisconsin, in front of him on the course, he had plenty of motivation. He finished in the middle of the pack on the bike ride, 1234th place. On the run, of 2081 competitors, there were only 110 who were faster.* ❧

 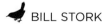

The Year of the Veterinarian

2011 has been designated "The Year of the Veterinarian." which struck me as a bit self-promotional. Is 2012 to be "The Year of the Vacuum Cleaner Salesman"?

As it turns out, the first veterinary college was formed in France, 250 years ago. At the time, diseases like Rinderpest were rampant, and could wipe out populations of horses over an entire continent. The first veterinarians were dedicated to preserving the health of livestock as well as public health and food safety. At the same time, veterinarians proposed that the study of animal disease and physiology could further our understanding of human medicine.

Today that dedication is no less intense. As our relationship with animals continues to evolve, the mission has come to include the advancement and protection of the human-animal bond.

While in the presence of veterinary professionals, I never fail to be impressed at the purity and sincerity of purpose, and the energy with which we pursue the advancement of animal health. It is a group I am intensely proud to belong to.

So when you bring your pet to us, we walk onto your farm, or you put a bite of safe food into your mouth, you can know there are 250 years of science and caring behind the service.

We are moved and motivated on a daily basis by you, the clients who care so much for your pets and work so hard for your herds. We appreciate you and we thank you. ◆

For the Love of a Cow

I hear a lot of talk about the food that families work to put on their tables. Many strive to buy "all natural." if not organic. Some literally snarl at the notion their 2% or skim may have originated from a FACTORY farm.

Agriculture in Wisconsin and this country employs tens of thousands of people and generates billions of dollars for our economy. I would ask that we consider the amazing quality of the product, and the daily dedication to the well-being of animals on large farms. Without dispute, few of us have more skills or work harder than a farmer. They wouldn't do it were it not for the Love of a Cow.

Thirty years ago, Dr. Stanley Curtis offered the concept of *The Welfare Plateau* to maximize productivity and animal husbandry. Simply put, the nicer we are to our cow, the more milk they make.

It is very much the focus of the dairy industry today. We seek to minimize stress by providing ideal areas to rest; fresh, dry air; plentiful, nutritious feed and clean water. Penmates who play nicely together make life more peaceful. Parlors are designed for easy entrance and exit. Milkers are selected for warm hands and soft voices.

Next time you pour a bowl of Corn Flakes,™ know that the milk is of the highest quality, produced by cows whose farmers still know many by name, and stop to scratch 'em on the head. ⬢

 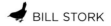 BILL STORK

Little Machine

My 14-year-old son, along with millions around the world, is holding his breath in anticipation of the release of the iPad 3.

For a fraction of the cost of a used Toyota, you can get a package of screen protectors, an "otter box" (recall 14-year-old son), extended no hassle service plan, 128 "gigs" of storage, and access to the world.

With an iPad, an imitation Stratocaster and a three-day weekend, you can learn to play Clapton, start a band, and record what used to be a record.

My friend Larry the Logger recently bought a brand-new, 30-year-old, four passenger plane. You guessed it — he found his way from the panhandle of Florida back home to Wyoming with an iPad. (So much for the seat of your pants.) Granted, his flight plan looked like the dotted line that follows Billy from Family Circus, but that's a Larry thing.

With more than a half-million apps, it's impossible to imagine the capabilities of this 8x8 device. The iPad is impressive by any measure, but by my way of thinking, feeble in comparison to my favorite machine, the wheelbarrow.

Created at least 2,500 years ago, you can still go to your local Ace Hardware and pick up Version 1.0 of the wheelbarrow any day of the week. History is not clear, but I am certain that lines were as long and hype as intense as the release of the IPad3. At 1/5 the price, you can get a contractor-grade workhorse in your choice of three colors, with pneumatic tire, fully assembled.

Let us try and quantify the value.

First, I went to my woodpile and gathered an armload that could be reasonably managed: 8 logs. The fireplace is only 40 meters (valid research is always metric) so I had to walk up the driveway and down the road until exhaustion, 100m.

Next, with the assistance of a compound lever and a 6ft³ bed, I was able to haul 40 logs. Sunday shoppers at the Piggly Wiggly looked twice at the guy effortlessly pushing a load of split oak around the parking lot. In the name of research, I remained focused. Final distance: 5km.

Having moved a load 5 times larger, 50 times farther, we have our conclusions. First, we are grateful the numbers were round. Second, we can multiply our output 50 times with a simple wheelbarrow. Our project was accomplished with entirely domestically manufactured products, using no fossil fuels, while getting great exercise.

From the Mayo Clinic to the Hoover Dam, there has never been a significant achievement in engineering and construction that has not used the mighty wheelbarrow. With no disrespect to the vision of the recently departed Steve Jobs, don't forget the simple stuff. ⬦

 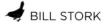

Mammas, Let Your Babies Grow Up...

The sun sets gold outside the little house on the hill. Inside, the air is saturated. The smell of Starbucks Espresso Roast singes the nostrils as Snooki whines of her latest crisis. Work clothes and shoes are hung neatly in the vestibule. A 4-oz bottle of formula sits on a column of *Wall Street Journal* as Jed and Jake nurse the two-week-old twins. Jake rattles a historic play-by-play of the storming of the Bastille, and how it launched the French Revolution.

The day is nearly done; the next is only hours away. By the time the sun warms the eastern sky, Jed, Jake and Rachel will be ready to roll. They'll climb into their handmade custom leather, and head to the office.

A typical day in corporate America, except their office is a 90,000-acre ranch in Wyoming. Jed, Jake and Rachel are Cowboys.

Their leather seat is a saddle, "custom" built to carry syringes and medicine to treat the 4,000 cattle they raise each year. They commute on Quarter Horses with names like Torque and Boomtruck. Many Rachel nurtured as foals and, after two years on the range, Jed and Jake saddled and rode. The twins they nursed are kid goats, and the work clothes in the vestibule are boots, buckles, spurs and lariats. The little house is 30 miles west on Horse Creek Road from the nearest pavement. It is a half tank of gas to get a gallon of 2% milk.

They are celebrated in song, romanticized in poems, photographed and painted. They are few and forgotten. They are Cowboys. Defined by the horse beneath their saddle and the cattle they save, they are as much a part of the land beneath their boots as the wells and windmills.

Innovate or die may apply in Silicon Valley, but here in Wyoming things have and will continue to be done the same for centuries. Horses from the Bartlett Ranch are sold to every corner of the continent, from kids in county fairs to team ropers and barrel racers. Their steers are sold to feedlots in the Front Range, and cows to graze on ranches in the Rockies.

Cowboys don't work for salaries, bonuses or promotions. Meet a cowboy on a fencing crew or working cattle in a chute, shirts will be tucked at their waist and buttoned at the wrist. They'll tip their hats and greet you with a "Pleasure, ma'am." What cowboys work for is also what defines them: stewardship of the land they love and animals they raise, and — more than anything else — pride. From the belt buckle, both ways. ⬦

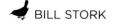 BILL STORK

R-E-S-P-E-C-T

She sat quietly in the far corner of the parking lot. Like Ike, a museum piece. Lee Iacocca's vision that launched a revolution: 29 years before on-board navigation and DVDs, it's the first generation minivan, with one sliding door, faux wood siding, running boards and three hubcaps.

Her pilot was an inspiration. At the Cambridge Piggly Wiggly, their dedication to hometown service is to carry your groceries to your car. It matters not if you are an Olympic powerlifter with one head of Romaine. The nice young folks are going to carry it to your car, make conversation and thank you for coming.

So when he emerged from the store, I had to smile. Past the pumpkins on the curb, his dress and his demeanor made it clear he belonged to the faded blue Grand Caravan. So as not to trouble anyone, he carried groceries on his right arm; on his left was his bride. Her hand under his, clasped just above the elbow, he walked cautiously a quarter step behind.

They rounded the grill and paused in unison as he found a dry spot on the blacktop to set the food, then turned to open her door. Like a slow waltz, he kept one hand on the door handle, the other on the small of her back. Once her coattails were safe and dry, he closed the door, stowed the groceries and headed home.

The nest has been empty for years. Yet, here is a man and woman who didn't have to reinvent husband and wife once their lives no longer revolved around baseball games and choir practice. Their children were raised by parents who loved one another unconditionally, supported without question, and respected those who served them.

We can do our children no greater service if we are to take a lesson from a little man in a mini-van on his way home from church, with his wife of 40 years. ❧

Forgiveness

Maybe you've read about him. Brian Banks is 26 years old, stands 6 feet 2 inches tall and weighs 245 lbs. He can lift a quarter of a ton, and run 40 yards in 4.6 seconds. Standing flat-footed, Brian can leap four and a half feet straight up or 10 feet across. Impressive feats of athleticism, but they speak nothing of his strength.

At 16, he was a standout linebacker at Long Beach Poly High School in San Diego California, with well-founded NFL aspirations. Among countless offers was a full ride scholarship to the University of Southern California. The summer before his senior year, it all evaporated. After a brief interlude with a classmate in a stairwell, Brian was accused of kidnapping and rape.

In 62 sworn statements he desperately maintained his innocence. Though there was not a shred of evidence to support the charges, his attorney advised him to plead no contest. History and the California court system were not on his side. His age, size and the color of his skin would all but guarantee a verdict and 40 years in prison. Reluctantly he pled, and was sentenced to six years.

After 62 months in jail, Brian was released. Branded a sex offender, he was fitted with a GPS bracelet and forbidden from schools, zoos and parks.

As proof that social media can do more than reunite college roommates, he received a "friend" request from the woman who had robbed him of youth and opportunity. With trepidation, fear and confusion, he replied. In two separate meetings, she would confess to fabricating the entire story, un-coerced, videotaped and in the presence of witnesses. On May 24th, all charges were dismissed. Brian bowed his head, cried, cut his bracelet and went to Sea World.

When freedom became a hope, Brian began to train like a man possessed. When it was a reality, six NFL teams offered him a chance. Reporters jumped the story with muscles flexed and guns blazing. They expected an angry man bent on vengeance. They found a man grateful for the opportunities before him.

 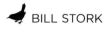 BILL STORK

With regard to the woman who took 10 years of his life, he is succinct and sincere: "If I allowed myself to be angry, I would be paralyzed. It's like when you're a little kid and mom tells you to clean your room. You get all mad for a while, but it doesn't get your room clean."

In a story dated June 18th, Seattle Seahawks coach Pete Carrol questions Bryan's conditioning and strength. I, for one, find it inspirational.

Epilogue: If Brian Banks never makes it to the NFL, you will probably never hear of him again. Sadly, the media largely missed the real story, by my way of thinking. The reason you probably haven't heard of Brian Banks before now is exactly why we should never forget him. ❧

To the Victor Go the Spoils

Michael Phelps punched the electronic pad at the end of his lane and cemented his place in history. In winning the Men's Individual 200m Medley, he became the most decorated Olympian of all time, and the greatest swimmer in history. Instantly was a message from President Obama. To follow will be magazine covers, Letterman, Leno and SNL, millions in endorsements, and thousands in prize money. Declaring he has swum his last race, the future is for him to choose.

Markus Deibler touched the same wall 0.71 seconds later. He pulled off his cap and goggles, stared stone-faced at the clock, caught his breath and climbed out of the pool. Race officials gave the 26-year-old German the equivalent of a British, "atta boy." Having finished in the top eight, he will receive a certificate of participation by mail. His English Wikipedia entry is one sentence (the German entry is a few paragraphs).

To be certain, either by physical prowess or an outright refusal to be defeated, Michael Phelps has something that other athletes do not. Equally certain is that, whether an Olympic gold medalist or an "also ran." every athlete with Olympic aspirations has sacrificed. An aspiring Olympic swimmer routinely averages 30 miles per week in the pool. As one put it, "I've been in pain so long, it's become just the way I feel."

To the victor go the spoils, as it has always been. While we recover from our Olympic hangover, there will be no forgetting Michael, Gabby, and Usain. At the same time, let us remember Markus, Mykola and Wilson. Whether the Olympics, or the shortstop on our little league team, let us consider no person who has done their best superior to another who can say the same. ✐

 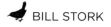 BILL STORK

Blessed are the Sick

Saint Lawrence Catholic Church is a house of worship and reflection. Perched atop one of southern Wisconsin's rolling drumlins, her steeple is visible from half the county. Through the stained glass windows drifts the fertile aroma of fresh plowed ground. Half a year later, crisp fall wind rattles the leaves of corn waiting for harvest.

I have no recollection what Father Tom said before or after, but when he quoted Mother Teresa, "Blessed are the sick," I froze bolt upright in my pew, left stone-cold still and reflective. Over months and miles to follow, I came to appreciate the profundity of those four words.

I watched Bob Leiner flatly deny terminal cancer. He had the transmission out of his daughter's car and promised to remodel his son's bathroom; it just wasn't his time yet. I saw neighbors come to his aid.

I saw friends, family, and perfect strangers circle the wagons and raise hope, support and thousands of dollars for a six-year-old girl with cancer, she and her family not having slept two consecutive hours in months.

I watched dementia erode my mother's clarity, as Dad stood silently behind her, for better or worse, in health and in sickness. Cooking and cleaning as she had for 50 years, he gave her all the credit and maintained her dignity at any cost.

Ah, yes, Mother T, blessed are the sick.

For Mom, the first sign of decline was that her handwriting on the cards she sent religiously was less than a work of art. Her chocolate chip cookies weren't as soft.

Aging is inevitable. Any attempts to deny it are likely to prove futile. ❧

Little John of God*

From the choir loft, one joyous voice fills the chapel and permeates every crevice with, "Hark the Herald Angels Sing," while below the flock shuffles in. Many have traveled for days, while others from just down the block. In the very first pew sit Elizabeth and Brian, their heads bowed in silent contemplation. Between them is Robby, legs swinging just short of touching the floor, contemplating the big square box under the tree at home.

Between Elizabeth and the aisle are 18 inches of empty pew, the only unoccupied space in the church. St. James Catholic Church has celebrated midnight mass for 125 years, yet it is the last place you would have found Elizabeth, were it not for a boy who never spoke a word, took a step, or fed himself a single bite of food.

Not long ago, Christmas Eve would have found Elizabeth on a bar stool, surrounded by cigarette smoke and honky-tonk, rather than incense and choir. Hungry for attention in any form, surrounded by disingenuous people disguised as friends, she would eventually find herself with a tortured soul, a gravid womb and choices.

In an ultimate demonstration of "that which doesn't kill you," Elizabeth found employment and reunited with her family. Months later, John was welcomed into the world by a mother and her parents who would always love him. Unconditional love would be put to the test, but never fail. As John grew older, Cerebral Palsy would rob him of the ability to walk, speak, or respond in a traditional way. In the face of it all, every Sunday morning would find them at St. James Catholic Church, John in his chair by the aisle, Elizabeth on his left, the only direction he could look.

Following Lenten service on a glorious March day, the recessional hymn poured through the open doors as Elizabeth loaded John into their van. A hand grazed her shoulder as a trembling voice asked, "Would you like to go for breakfast?"

She turned to see Brian, raised her eyebrows, looked to John and back again. Brian more than understood. In the month of Sundays

 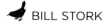 BILL STORK

it had taken him to summon the courage to approach Elizabeth, he had watched them. Always patient, never apologizing, she spoke to John as a young man. Of everything she provided, the most important was dignity. John, in turn, provided the same for her.

Surprised by the invitation, she smiled and nodded, "we would like that." John had helped Elizabeth turn the corner. Now he had helped her find a man who, from that day forward and to the present, would show her the respect she had found in herself. In time they would wed, and together welcome Robby into their family.

At Christmas we celebrate the birth of Jesus Christ. Regardless of how our faith may fall there are people who have helped us become whole and strong; perhaps our parents, a perfect stranger or Jesus Christ. For Elizabeth, it was a boy who didn't live to his tenth birthday.

Let us take this opportunity to recognize those who are inseparably woven into who we are, embrace our roles in the lives of children, and appreciate the beauty and strength of others.

Merry Christmas!

The title of this article is borrowed from a song of the same name, performed by the venerable Latino folk and rock band, Los Lobos. Humbly calling themselves, "just another band from East L.A.," the last 40 years have proven they are anything but. The song has been covered, and re-recorded countless times, but originally appeared on 'The Neighborhood'. Of this simple song that very much reflects the sentiment of this article, several versions, including a duet with Emmy Lou Harris, are readily available on YouTube. ❧

Swing Low

As I sit with my coffee in the glow of our Christmas tree, my thoughts cannot be kept from New Town, Connecticut. I had intended to specifically not write about the unspeakable horror that took place there. However, any attempt to direct a meaningful thought anywhere else was futile.

Attempt for a moment to internalize the grief of the families who lost loved ones, and the fiscal cliff, the drought, the stock market, and the Super Bowl become inconsequential. I can only hope that every last one of us is in some meaningful way affected.

In tribute and memory of the innocent victims, our space in the newspaper this week will be left intentionally blank. ⬥

 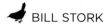

Silent Night

December 24th, 1942, a small town in central England. Catholics filed into church for midnight mass, silent in reverence; dark in order to survive. Outside, WWII raged; towns went black at night to avoid air raids. Six pews remained conspicuously vacant. Just before midnight the giant cathedral doors creaked open. One by one they shambled in, pausing to touch fingers to the Holy Water and cross themselves. Chained and shackled, German and Italian POWs were led by armed guards down the aisle. They shuffled into the empty seats.

As the priest welcomed the congregation, he announced there would be no music, as the organist had fallen ill. With the world consumed in conflict, midnight mass was perhaps the only thing villagers could look forward to. Parishioners breathed a collective sigh. Just then a German prisoner whispered to his guard. The guard tilted his chin, and approached the altar. The priest nodded.

The guard led the prisoner to the organ and dropped the chains. The prisoner took the bench, laid his mangled hands on the keys, dropped his head, and began. As if a foretelling of peace that would take years to achieve, he played with passion, conviction and grace. Allied voices joined the German's chords in a crescendo that rose through the bell tower to fill cobbled streets below.

This story was retold on Christmas Day, 2012, in Cambridge, Wisconsin. I daresay that regardless of one's race or religion, the message remains the same: two groups of people divided by a war that killed millions, came together as one. To be certain, enormous conflict still exists around the globe, but we have cleaned up some big scuffles. As Christmas and New Year fade to a dot in our rearview mirror, let us resolve to do what we can right here in Jefferson County, Wisconsin.

Tolerance is defined as a fair, objective and permissive attitude towards others who may believe differently than us. A fine and admirable goal, yet one that I find historic and inadequate. Let us "goo gone" the stickers off our bumpers and replace them with "Embrace: to take in or include as a more inclusive whole."

Happy New Year.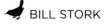

BILL STORK

Beautiful Music

I have sat two tables away from Kristy Larson, slack-jawed and stupid as she dropped the final "I'm so lonesome I could cry." in homage to her painfully early departed brother. I have been paralyzed as Alison Krauss stood solo, stomped, crooned and built "Down to the River to Pray," from the Olde Town School of Folk Music stage, to the heavens. I have clenched and trembled as Susan Tedeschi growled from her diaphragm "how in the hell can a person go to work in the morning, come home in the evening, and have nothing to say."

Though I have heard music more beautiful, I have never been so inspired as at Christmas morning Mass.

The Christmas crowd stomped snow and shuffled in. As Father Dave opened his arms wide and welcomed the flock, the holiday din faded to mute.

Silent may have been the night; morning not so much. Throughout the first and second reading, all that could be heard were pages of the missalette. But Cheerios, big plastic car keys, and "pass the baby" only last so long. By the homily, the youngest of the congregation began a choir of their own.

As gifts were prepared, kneelers dull-thudded against the carpet, and back against their pegs as we all filed down the aisle to receive communion. Against the rhythmic moan of the organ, heads down and hands crossed, we waddled toward the Altar. The murmur of "Body of Christ" and "Amen" were all that could be heard.

As the last row accepted the host, crossed themselves, and returned to their pews, the joy of the day could no longer be contained.

With a tremble in her hands she caressed the keys. With pitch not quite perfect, she projected to the heavens a heartfelt Hallelujah. Last in line to receive the host, with the gait of a soldier returning from war and his right sleeve hanging empty, Phil took his place next to the organ. He joined voice with Beth, and with a mighty silver jingle raised the traditional Christmas tambourine. With that, the congregation joined and swelled in full voice.

It is nearly a new year, a time when folks are prone to resolve. Speaking for myself, I was moved to the core by Beth and Phil. A fraction of their faculties may have fallen casualty to blood clots and corn pickers, yet their soul, faith and spirit were only amplified.

Whether January 1 or July 17, let us take whatever physical, mental and spiritual strength we can muster to be as productive, kind and benevolent as humanly possible. ◈

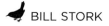 BILL STORK

Giving Thanks

Above my desk hangs a plaque:

" I solemnly swear to use my scientific knowledge and skills for the benefit of society through the protection of animal health, the relief of animal suffering, the conservation of livestock resources, the promotion of public health, and the advancement of medical knowledge."

The Veterinarian's Oath has guided our profession for 150 years.

The thread that binds us as vets is that we get to work with and for people who care deeply about animals. On farms in the production sense, where the better environment and feed we provide, the healthier and more productive the herd. In the companion animal paradigm, we meet all types of people. Regardless who they are Monday through Friday and how they may be perceived at large, as veterinarians, we see them caring for their animals.

We have known...

...the stray lab who would not leave the side of a young boy in a wheelchair, and the owner who tracked grass clippings into the clinic from working odd jobs to pay his bill,

...the terrier who will not rest a wink until every squirrel, rabbit and stray cat is in a tree, a hole, or Dodge County, and who also will not leave the lap of a boy with Autism.

There is a lady nearly eighty years old, long widowed, all the while supported by her daughters, who has defeated three separate cancers. Her cats, Orville and Melvin, need her.

There are the farmers, with skill sets born of necessity — if not survival — who are bound first and foremost by the value of family. They are stewards of this land, unspeakably beautiful, muscular, and productive. Whether tens or hundreds, every dairy farm I have ever set boots on still has cows with names, and men who cry when they die.

As we approach the last Thursday of November, we at the Lake Mills Veterinary Clinic are thankful for our patients and clients, many of whom have become friends. We are grateful to be a part of their care. They teach us on a daily basis the inherent good in people, as they care for their animals. Many have inspired us professionally and grown us personally. ⬦

 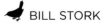

About the Author

Dr. Bill Stork grew up in a meat and potatoes, git-'er-done, Mr. and Mrs., "In the name of the Father..." household in Decatur, Illinois. Population 100,000 and shrinking. He attended public schools at a time when racial tensions and desegregation were a fact of life. He came home to after-school snacks from a stay-at-home mother. His dad worked construction. Unless Dad worked overtime, Bill and his parents — and frequently neighbors needing help welding or with a carburetor they needed help rebuilding — would sit down at the table. Bread was broken, thanks were given and days were discussed. If his homework was done and dishes clean, secondary education commenced at the work bench, vice and welder.

The first manifestation of his love for animals came in kindergarten when the family insurance salesman invited the family to look at a litter of collie puppies. "Sugar" was lonely in the basement, so Little Bill dragged his blanket and pillow down the steps and slept on the concrete until she was brave enough to spend the night alone.

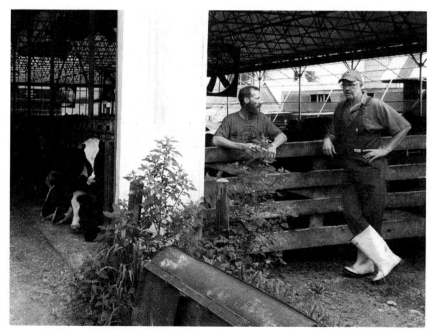

He first dreamed of writing while watching *The Waltons* on Thursday nights at age seven. He mowed lawns, walked beans, and helped neighbors paint and roof beginning at age 12, and landed a job at the Brush College Animal Hospital two years later. Six years of cleaning cages and scrubbing baseboards only served to fuel the fire ignited by reading James Herriot's *All Creatures Great and Small* for an 8th grade book report.

Dr. Stork was sheltered, in the sense that he grew up in the geographic and metaphorical center of the state and country. An hour down Interstate 72 and a bit farther than the apron strings could stretch, he attended the University of Illinois beginning in the fall of 1983. His sphere began to expand, and in the years to follow he would co-evolve in the likeness of friends who have since become brothers. They hailed from Chicago to Bombay, and were diverse in ethnicity, race and religion. They were common in the sense that their families were core.

He graduated from the University of Illinois – College of Veterinary Medicine in May 1992 and migrated across the Cheddar Curtain. In doing so, he surrendered the gratuitous use of "r's" (warsh the car), hardened his consonants and stretched out his "o's" (anybody using the boooat?). Intact was his record and CD collection and love of old school blues, country, folk and bluegrass music. On June 15th, 1992, he started working at the Lake Mills Veterinary Clinic. According to the Bank of Lake Mills, he can retire at or near age 125. When Brett Favre trotted on to replace the injured Don Majkowski, a hard core Packers Fan stood where a lukewarm Bears fan once did.

He currently shares a 7-acre petting zoo with a displaced Wyoming cattle dog, an aging Labrador, 2 goats, a cat named Stinker and 3 others, 11 horses and his one-person support crew and partner of 5 years, Sheila.

He is addicted to sunsets. Most of what you read was conceived on country roads and composed at or near sunrise. He is wholly uncomfortable writing about himself in the third person. ❧

 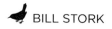

Acknowledgements

I have dreamed of writing a book since the age of 12. I watched the Waltons, entertained what seemed to be novel thoughts, and wrote in my diary. In college, I shared a pint or two with my friend Hal Leonard. At the resolution of each of the world's problems I would conclude with, "You know Harry, life is simple." Meeting adjourned. I promised Hal 25 years ago I would name the book after our tag line, but market research suggests we use James Herriot in the title.

The book would assuredly have remained a dream were it not for the OCD Behaviorist behind the screen. It is no exaggeration to say that were it not for the technical skill, tolerance, patience and sensitivity of my editor Mittsy Voiles, not a word would ever be written, published, or printed.

For someone who does not claim to be a writer, first you must step outside yourself and get comfortable "putting yourself out there." No two have been more supportive than Don and Mary Grant.

It is equally true that this would have never become a reality were it not for my partner Sheila Barnes. Whether our relationship is 'til death do us part, or tomorrow, my mind has been freed of need for companionship. My time has been liberated to create as I can, without guilt. I am immeasurably stronger thanks to my time with her.

I hope and pray that every one of us is blessed with a sacred group of friends and family. People come into our lives with a variety of upbringings, with unique attributes and strengths. Thanks in some part to character and chronology, they become part of our DNA. Every experience we have from the day we meet them is altered in a meaningful way. To name them is to risk omission, and obligate me to write another book. To not would be remiss. They are: Kishan Khemani, Scott R. Clewis, Gary Edmonds, Ned and Sarah Healy, Ryan Haack, Dr. William VanAlstine, Dr. Arlin Rodgers, Dr. Rand Gustafson, Barb, and Sheila Mathwig.

I have known Glenn Fuller since minutes after arriving in Wisconsin. He has helped me through every kind of tough time. Glenn is the friend you know is there. This book could have been written in half the time, but, hoping that these words might be wrapped in a cover of his design, I have agonized to assemble words and build images that are worthy of his art.

Though many came before him, it's never been done better: espousing family values, Michael Perry has re-validated heartland poetry. His coming-home novel, *Population 485*, is the book I had intended to write. He proved it could be done, and has made himself accessible to us wanna-bes. This dream would not have come to fruition without him.

To live in the hearts of those you leave behind is to not die. As a result, The Amazing Dick Bass is immortal and typing his name brings tears.

I thank my son Calvin and daughter Paige for surrendering their anonymity and keeping me centered. ◅◈▻

 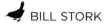 BILL STORK